I0842271

AGE SLOWER,

LIVE LONGER

A Guide to Longevity and Vitality

Howard Henry

Copyright © 2023 Howard Henry

All rights reserved. No part of this book may be reproduced in any form or by any electronic or mechanical means, including information storage and retrieval systems, without permission in writing from the publisher, except by a reviewer who may quote brief passages in a review.

This book is intended for general information purposes only. It is not intended to provide medical, legal, or other professional advice. The information contained in this book is provided without any express or implied warranties. Every effort has been made to ensure accuracy, but the author and publisher make no representations or warranties of any kind with regard to the accuracy, completeness, or the suitability of the information contained herein for any purpose.

TABLE OF CONTENTS

Introduction to Longevity and Vitality

Longevity and vitality are two key concepts that are essential for a long and healthy life.

Longevity refers to the length of one's life, while vitality is the quality of life. To achieve longevity and vitality, it is necessary to maintain a lifestyle that is conducive to both physical and mental health. This includes a healthy diet, regular physical activity, adequate sleep, stress management, and an overall positive outlook. Additionally, managing chronic conditions, such as heart disease and diabetes, is key to maintaining longevity and vitality. By following these strategies, individuals can improve their longevity and vitality, while also significantly reducing the risk of developing serious illnesses.

By understanding the importance of longevity and vitality, individuals can make informed decisions about their health. Knowledge of lifestyle changes that can improve these two components of health can lead to improved overall well-being. Additionally, being aware of medical conditions that can affect longevity and vitality can help individuals make proactive decisions for the future. Ultimately, maintaining longevity and vitality can help individuals live a longer, healthier and more vibrant life.

The goal of this book is to provide an introduction to longevity and vitality, as well as how to achieve them. Through understanding the importance of both, individuals can make informed decisions about their health and lifestyle choices.

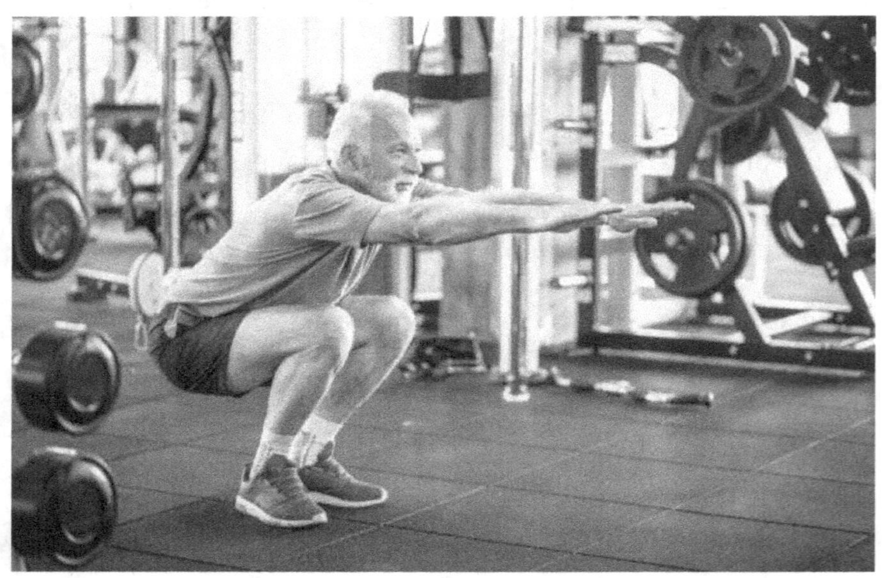

A TESTIMONY OF LIFE LIVED TO THE FULNESS

Robert had just celebrated his 110th birthday, and the doctors were amazed by his sound health. He had outlived his peers by several decades, and his longevity had become a source of wonder for many.

Robert had been born into a family of modest means, but he had worked hard all his life to make sure that he and his family were well provided for. He had worked in a variety of jobs, including farming, construction, and factory work. He had also done some teaching in the local school.

But despite all the hard work, Robert had always kept a healthy lifestyle. He ate healthy, home-cooked meals every day and exercised regularly. He also took time each day to meditate and practice yoga. He had always been an early riser, and he still rose at 4:30 every morning for a brisk walk and some stretching.

Robert never smoked, drank alcohol or ate junk food. He drank plenty of water and got plenty of rest. He also took regular supplements, such as fish oil and vitamin D, to keep his body functioning properly.

As a result, Robert had managed to keep his body healthy and strong despite his advanced age. He had no major health problems and still had all his teeth at 110. His vision and hearing were still good, and he had few aches and pains.

Robert also had a positive attitude that had kept him going all these years. He was grateful for every day he had been given, and he looked forward to the future with optimism. Robert was an avid reader and enjoyed learning new things. He was also an artist, and he loved to express himself through painting and drawing.

Robert also had a deep faith that had kept him going through the years. He prayed regularly and believed in the power of the divine to bring peace and joy into his life. He was also a big believer in the power of forgiveness, and he was always ready to forgive and forget.

Robert's life was a testament to the power of healthy living, positive thinking and lifestyle. He was an inspiration to all who knew him, and his example was one that everyone should strive to emulate. Robert was an amazing man, and there was no doubt that he was doing something right to have lived to such a ripe old age and remain so sound and healthy. No matter how old you are. Robert's example was one that everyone should strive to emulate and his life was a reminder that it is never too late to start.

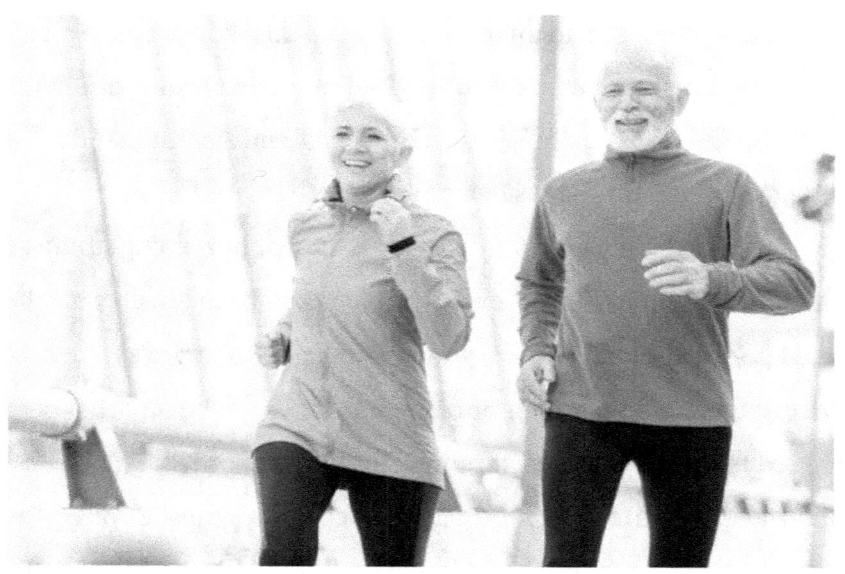

CHAPTER ONE

Nutrition for Longevity

Nutrition is an essential factor in achieving longevity. Good nutrition helps to ensure that our bodies are adequately supplied with essential nutrients to maintain good health and support our overall well-being. Eating a balanced diet that is rich in essential vitamins and minerals, as well as macronutrients such as proteins, carbohydrates, and fats, can help to promote healthy aging and increase longevity.

It is important to include a variety of foods in our diet to ensure that we are getting all the necessary nutrients. Eating a wide variety of fruits and vegetables, whole grains, and lean proteins is a great way to provide our bodies with the nutrients it needs. In addition, we should limit our intake of processed and refined foods, as these are often low in nutritional value.

It is also important to ensure that our bodies are adequately supplied with essential fatty acids. These can be found in fish, nuts, seeds, and vegetable oils, and are important for maintaining a healthy heart, brain, and immune system.

It is also important to stay hydrated. Drinking plenty of water throughout the day helps to keep our bodies functioning optimally. Staying hydrated also helps to flush out toxins and keep our skin looking healthy and youthful.

An essential element of a healthy lifestyle is exercise. Regular exercise helps to keep our bones and muscles strong and can help to reduce the risk of many chronic illnesses.

By following a healthy diet and exercising regularly, we can promote longevity and ensure that our bodies are in optimal condition for years to come. Eating a balanced diet and maintaining an active lifestyle are essential steps that we can take to ensure that we are living a long and healthy life.

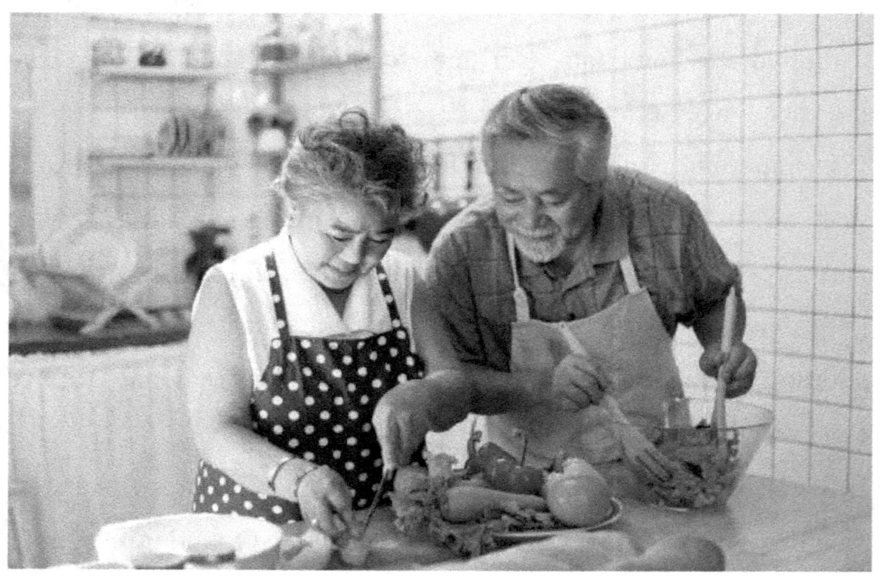

The classes of foods that promote longevity are nutrient-dense foods that are high in vitamins, minerals, antioxidants, and fiber. These include fruits, vegetables, whole grains, legumes, nuts, seeds, and quality proteins such as fish, poultry, and lean red meats. Eating a diet rich in these foods helps to reduce the risk of chronic diseases and can lead to a longer life.

Fruits and vegetables are packed with vitamins, minerals, and antioxidants that help fight free radicals that can damage cells and lead to diseases. Eating a variety of fruits and vegetables can help to increase your intake of essential vitamins and minerals and reduce your risk of developing chronic diseases.

Whole grains provide essential vitamins, minerals, and fiber. Eating whole grains can help to lower cholesterol, reduce inflammation, and reduce the risk of developing diabetes, heart disease, and some cancers.

Legumes are a fantastic source of fiber, vitamins, and minerals as well as plant-based protein. Consuming beans can lower cholesterol, enhance digestion, and lower your risk of getting some cancers.

Healthy fats, protein, vitamins, and minerals can all be found in large quantities in nuts and seeds. Eating a variety of nuts and seeds can help to reduce inflammation, lower cholesterol, and improve heart health.

Quality proteins such as fish, poultry, and lean red meats provide essential amino acids and minerals. Eating lean proteins can help to improve muscle growth, reduce inflammation, and reduce the risk of developing certain types of cancer.

Including these nutrient-dense foods in your diet can help to promote longevity and reduce the risk of developing chronic diseases. Eating a variety of these foods can help to ensure that you get all of the essential vitamins, minerals, fibers, and proteins that your body needs.

20 Examples Of Fruits And Vegetables

1. Apple – A round, sweet fruit with a crunchy texture, apple is a popular snack and can be cooked in a variety of ways.

2. Banana – Long, curved yellow fruit with a sweet taste, often eaten raw or in smoothies and desserts.

3. Orange – A citrus fruit with a juicy, tart flavor that can be enjoyed fresh, juiced, or in baked goods.

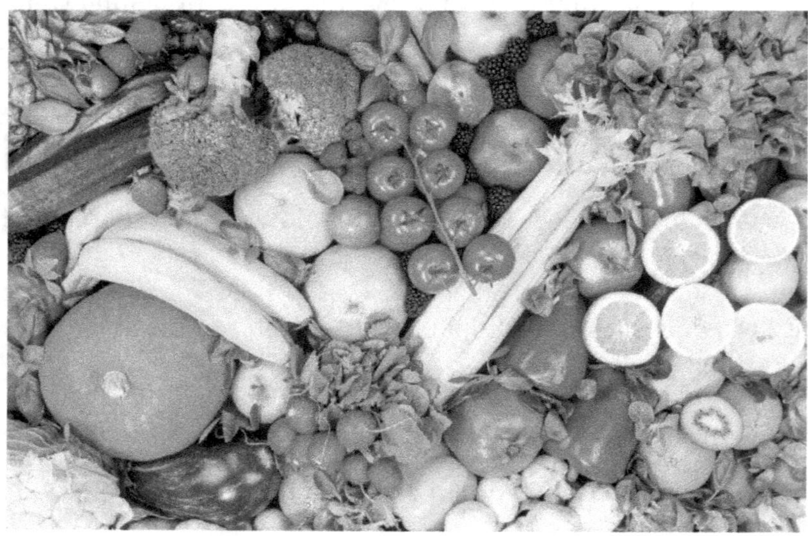

4. Grapefruit – A large, tart citrus fruit that can be eaten raw or juiced for a refreshing drink.

5. Strawberry – A small, sweet red berry with a juicy texture, often eaten fresh or in desserts.

6. Blueberry – A small, sweet dark blue berry with a tart flavor, often eaten fresh or in muffins.

7. Mango – A large, sweet yellow fruit with a juicy texture, often enjoyed fresh or as a smoothie.

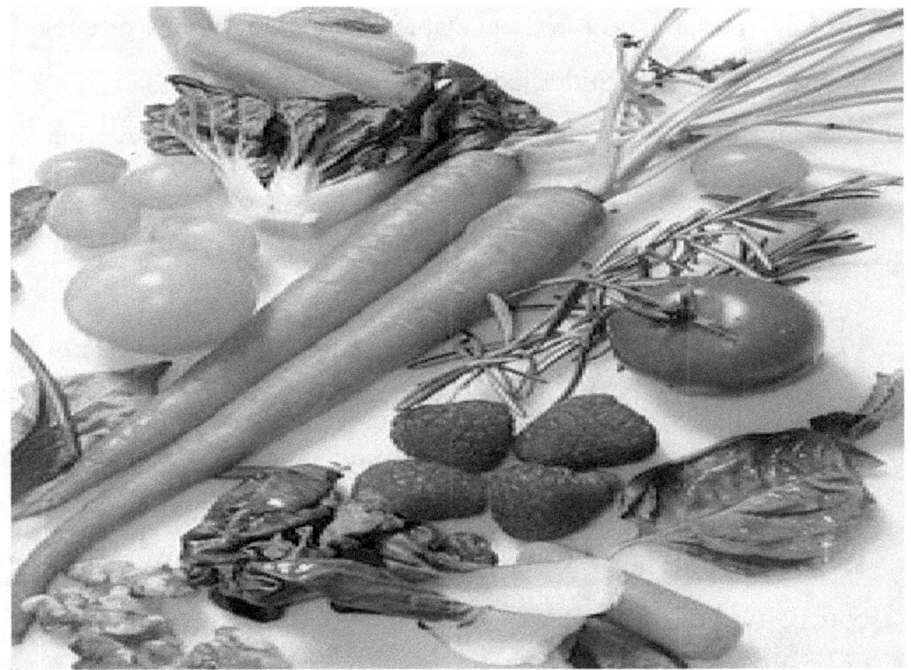

8. Watermelon – A large, sweet pink fruit with a crunchy texture, often enjoyed fresh or as a juice.

9. Pineapple – A large, sweet yellow fruit with a spiky texture, often eaten fresh or in smoothies.

10. Carrot – A crunchy orange vegetable, often enjoyed raw or cooked in dishes like soup and stir-fry.

11. Broccoli – A crunchy green vegetable, often enjoyed raw or cooked in dishes like casseroles and salads.

12. Spinach – A leafy green vegetable, often enjoyed raw or cooked in dishes like omelettes and quiches.

13. Lettuce – A light green vegetable, often enjoyed raw in salads or cooked in dishes like tacos and burritos.

14. Beetroot – A deep red vegetable, often enjoyed raw or cooked in dishes like soups and salads.

15. Potato – A starchy white vegetable, often enjoyed boiled, mashed, or fried in dishes like chips and hashbrowns.

16. Onion – A crunchy white vegetable, often enjoyed raw or cooked in dishes like stews and curries.

17. Cucumber – A crunchy green vegetable, often enjoyed raw in salads or cooked in dishes like stir-fry and soup.

18. Tomato – A juicy red vegetable, often enjoyed raw in salads or cooked in dishes like pasta and pizza.

19. Sweet Potato – A starchy orange vegetable, often enjoyed boiled, mashed, or roasted in dishes like casseroles.

20. Peas – A sweet green vegetable, often enjoyed raw or cooked in dishes like risottos and pies.

EATING FOR A HEALTHY HEART

Eating for a healthy heart is essential for overall health and well-being. A healthy diet can help reduce the risk of heart disease, stroke, and other chronic conditions. Eating foods that are high in fiber, low in saturated fat, and rich in omega-3 fatty acids can help reduce cholesterol levels, improve blood pressure, and reduce inflammation.

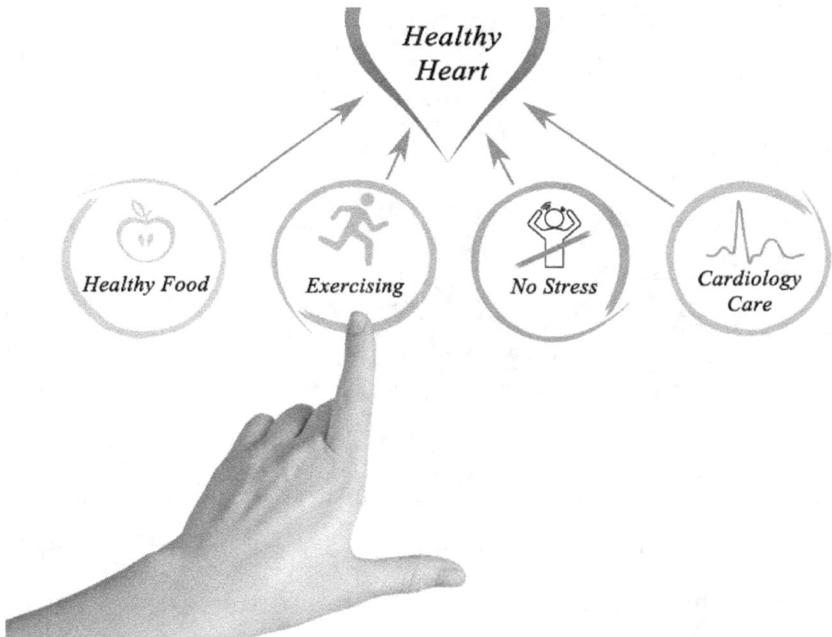

Fruits and vegetables are an important part of a healthy diet, as they are packed with vitamins and minerals, and are low in saturated fat. Eating five servings of fruits and vegetables each day is recommended by most health experts. Additionally, whole grains are an excellent source of fiber, which helps reduce cholesterol and improve blood pressure. Eating two to three servings of whole grains each day can help promote good heart health.

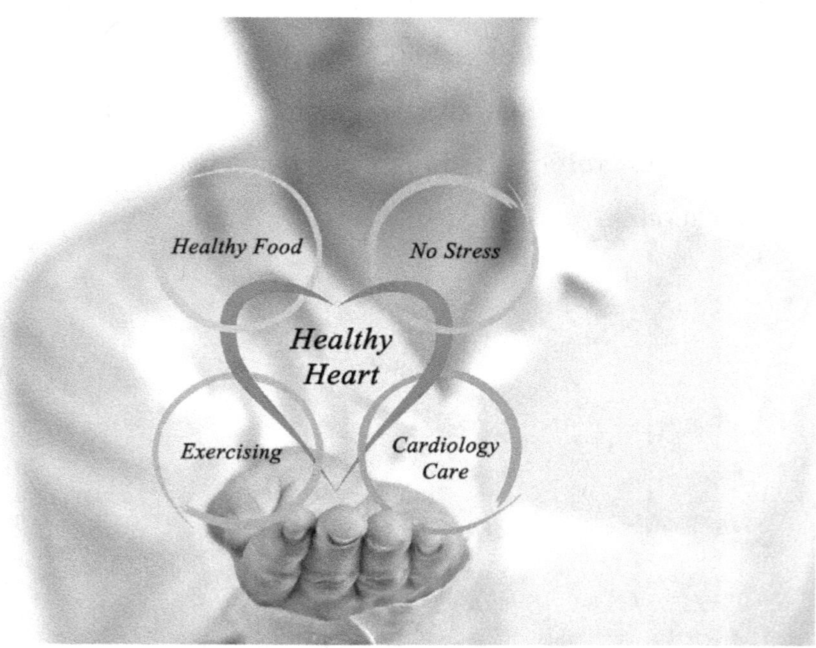

In addition to eating a healthy diet, it is important to limit the amount of salt and processed foods consumed. Too much salt can increase blood pressure, while processed foods are often high in trans fats, which increase the risk of heart disease.

Finally, regular physical activity can help keep the heart healthy. Exercise helps improve circulation, increases the heart's efficiency, and helps reduce cholesterol levels. Attempt to engage in physical activity most days of the week for at least 30 minutes.

Eating for a healthy heart is not only important for overall health and well-being, but can also reduce the risk of heart disease, stroke, and other chronic conditions. By eating a balanced diet that is high in fiber, low in saturated fat, and rich in omega-3 fatty acids, and getting regular physical activity, you can help keep your heart healthy for years to come.

EATING FOR A HEALTHY BRAIN

Maintaining the health of your brain requires eating a balanced diet. Eating a balanced diet that is high in fruits, vegetables, whole grains, and lean protein can help fuel your brain and keep it functioning at its best.

Fruits and vegetables are packed with vitamins and minerals that can help protect your brain from cognitive decline. Eating a variety of fruits and vegetables can also help keep your heart healthy, which is important for good circulation and brain health. Whole grains like oats, quinoa, and brown rice are rich in B vitamins, which are important for brain health. Eating a diet rich in whole grains can help reduce your risk of developing dementia and other age-related cognitive decline.

Lean proteins like fish, poultry, and legumes are also important for brain health. Fish is high in omega-3 fatty acids, which are essential for brain development and function. Eating a variety of lean proteins can help keep your brain healthy and protect it from age-related decline.

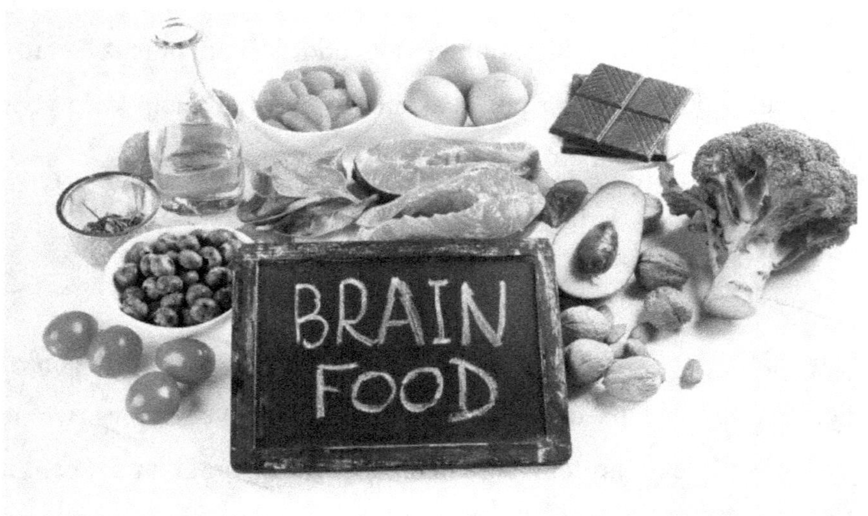

Staying well hydrated is also essential for brain health. Dehydration can lead to increased fatigue, difficulty concentrating, and impaired cognitive function. Drinking plenty of water throughout the day can help keep your brain functioning optimally. In addition to eating a healthy diet, getting regular physical activity is important for brain health. Exercise increases blood flow to the brain and can help improve cognitive function. Moreover, it can assist with stress relief and mood enhancement. By eating a healthy diet and getting regular physical activity, you can help keep your brain healthy and functioning optimally.

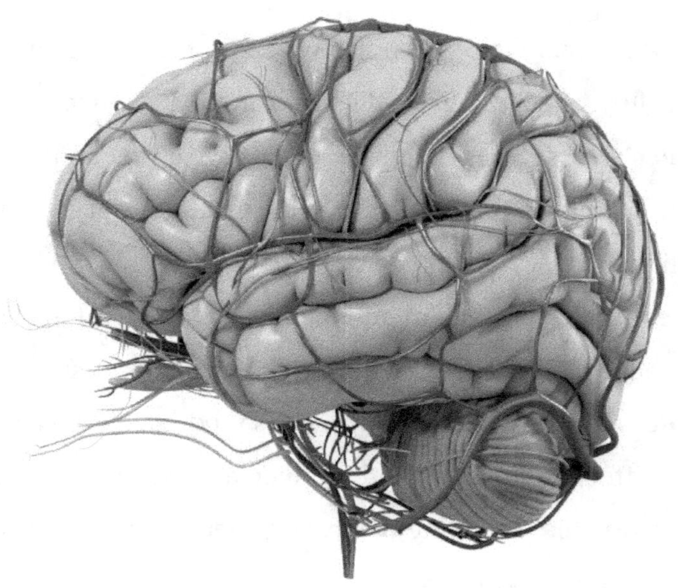

10 Simple Ways To Keep The Brain Healthy

1. Exercise regularly: Regular physical exercise increases blood flow to the brain, which helps the brain to function more efficiently.

2. Get enough sleep: Sleep is essential for the brain to recharge and process information.

3. Eat a healthy diet: Eating a diet rich in fruits, vegetables, and whole grains helps to keep the brain healthy and can help reduce the risk of dementia.

4. Challenge your mind: Doing puzzles, playing games, and learning new skills can help keep the brain active and healthy.

5. Socialize: Socializing with friends and family can help keep the brain healthy, as it stimulates the mind and helps reduce stress.

6. Reduce stress: Stress can have a negative effect on the brain, so it is important to find ways to reduce stress, such as yoga or meditation.

7. Take breaks: Taking regular breaks throughout the day can help to reduce stress and give the brain a chance to rest.

8. Avoid drugs and alcohol: Drugs and alcohol can have a negative effect on the brain and can increase the risk of dementia.

9. Stay hydrated: Drinking plenty of water helps to keep the brain healthy and functioning properly.

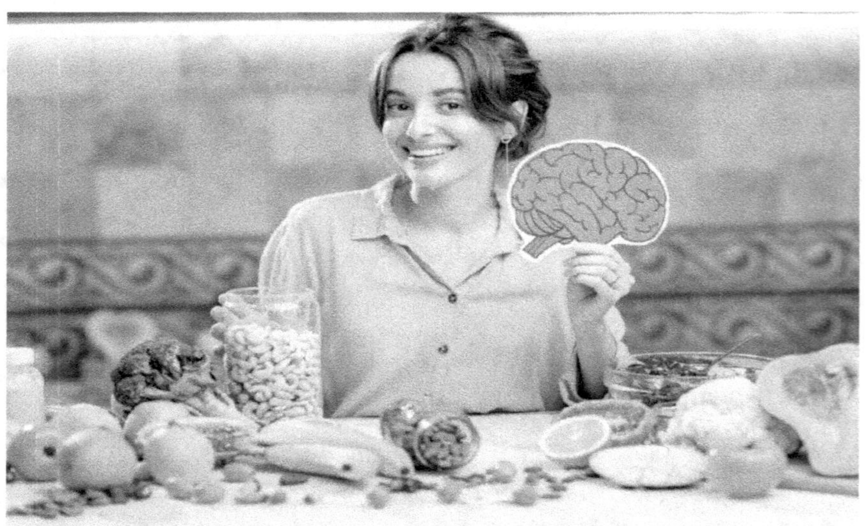

10. Manage your time: Balancing work and leisure activities can help to reduce stress and give the brain a chance to rest.

FOODS TO AVOID

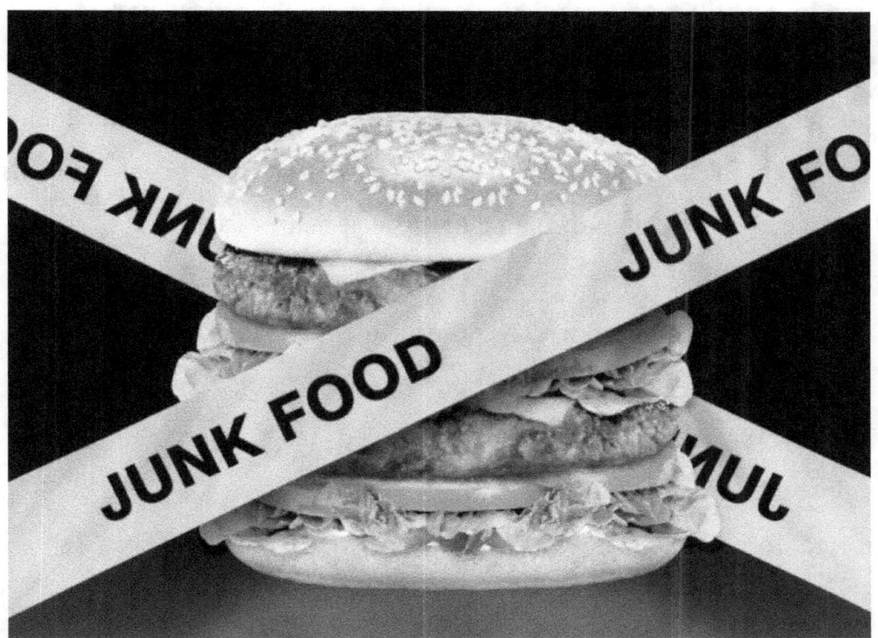

A long and healthy life depends heavily on eating a good diet. While there is no single one-size-fits-all diet that is suitable for everyone, there are some foods that should be avoided in order to maximize longevity. The following foods should be avoided in order to live a long life.

Processed meats, such as bacon, sausage, and ham, are high in saturated fat and sodium, both of which have been linked to increased risk of heart disease and stroke. Additionally, processed meats have been linked to increased risk of certain cancers, such as colon cancer. Processed meats are also high in preservatives and additives, which can be damaging to health.

Refined carbohydrates, such as white bread, pasta, and white rice, are low in fiber and can cause a spike in blood sugar levels. These refined carbohydrates can also lead to weight gain and an increased risk of type 2 diabetes. Whole grains, on the other hand, are high in fiber and can help to improve blood sugar control, reduce cholesterol, and reduce the risk of heart disease.

Sugary drinks, such as soda, energy drinks, and fruit juices, are high in sugar and calories. These drinks can lead to weight gain, increased risk of diabetes, and can damage teeth. Water is the best option for hydration, but unsweetened tea and coffee can be consumed in moderation.

Fried foods, such as french fries and fried chicken, are high in saturated fat, which can increase cholesterol levels and risk of heart disease. Baked, grilled, and steamed foods are better options for a healthy diet.

Red and processed meats, such as beef, pork, and processed meats, are high in saturated fat and can increase the risk of heart disease and certain cancers. Leaner meats, such as chicken and fish, are healthier alternatives.

Salt is an essential component of a healthy diet but should be consumed in moderation. Too much salt can increase blood pressure and lead to an increased risk of stroke and heart disease.

Another substance that needs to be taken in moderation is alcohol.. Regular alcohol consumption can increase the risk of certain cancers, liver damage, and high blood pressure.

In order to live a long life, it is important to be mindful of what you eat. Avoiding the above foods can help to reduce the risk of certain chronic diseases and maximize longevity. Eating a balanced diet with plenty of fruits, vegetables, whole grains, and healthy proteins is the best way to ensure a healthy, long life.

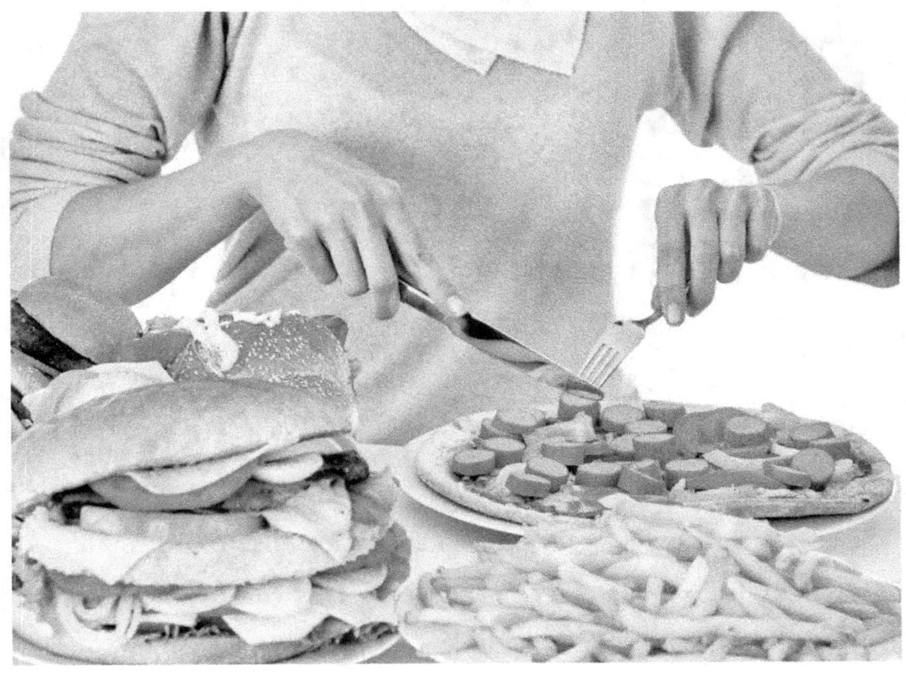

CHAPTER TWO

EXERCISE FOR LONGEVITY

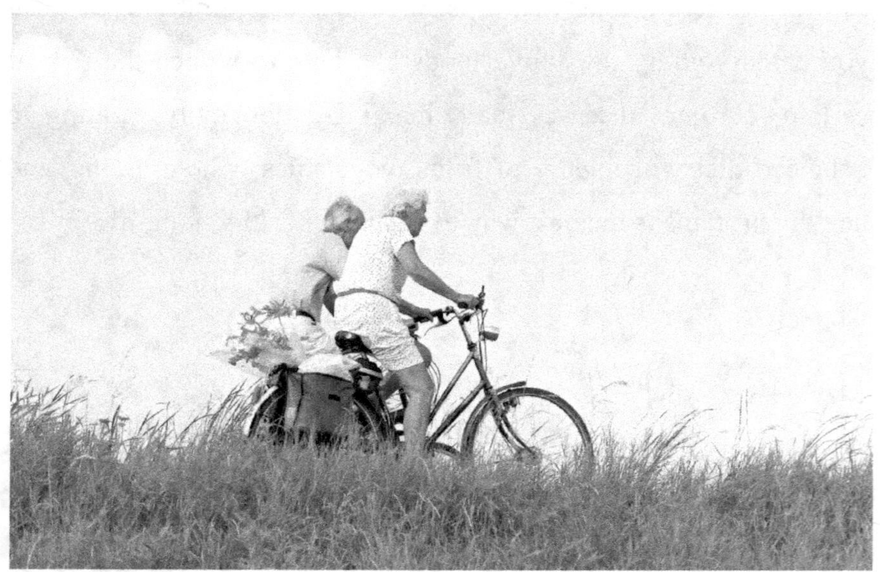

Exercise is one of the best things you can do for your body and your overall health, including your longevity. Regular exercise helps your body stay strong, fit, and healthy and can even help slow down the aging process.

The American Heart Association recommends that adults get at least 150 minutes of moderate intensity exercise or 75 minutes of vigorous intensity exercise each week. This can include a variety of activities such as walking, jogging, biking, swimming, or strength training.

In addition to the recommended amount of physical activity, there are several other things you can do to help promote longevity. Regularly stretching or practicing yoga can help keep your muscles and joints flexible and reduce the risk of injury. Getting enough rest is also important as it helps your body recover and recharge. Eating a balanced diet full of nutrient-rich foods can also help support a healthy lifestyle.

Exercise is an important part of a healthy lifestyle and can help promote longevity. Incorporating regular physical activity into your routine, along with healthy eating habits, can help you live a longer, healthier life.

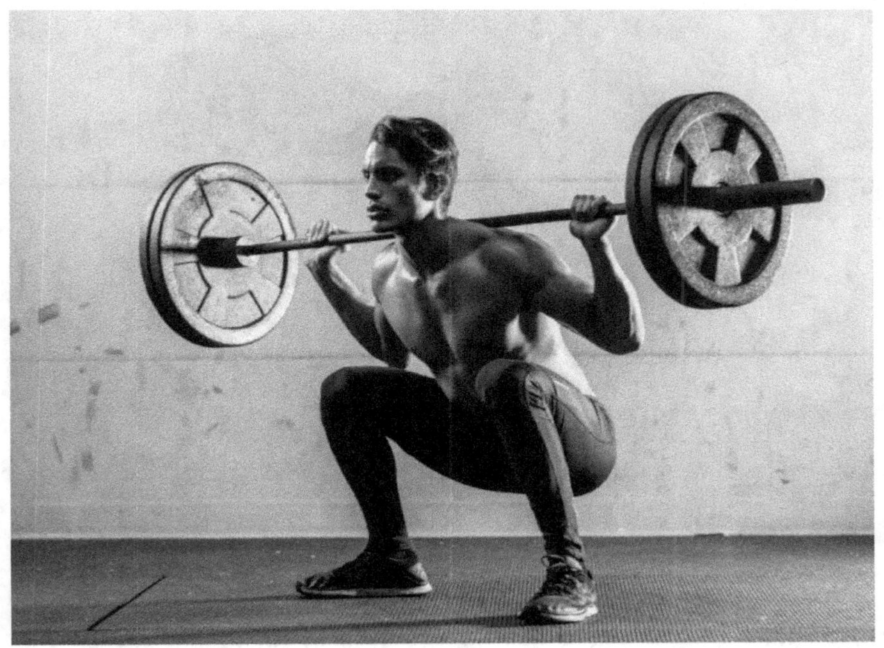

STRENGTH TRAINING

Strength training is a form of physical exercise that focuses on developing muscular strength and power. It involves a variety of exercises and activities that target the muscles of the body and use resistance to improve muscular strength, endurance, and power. Strength training can include a variety of exercises such as weightlifting, bodyweight exercises, plyometrics, and other forms of resistance training.

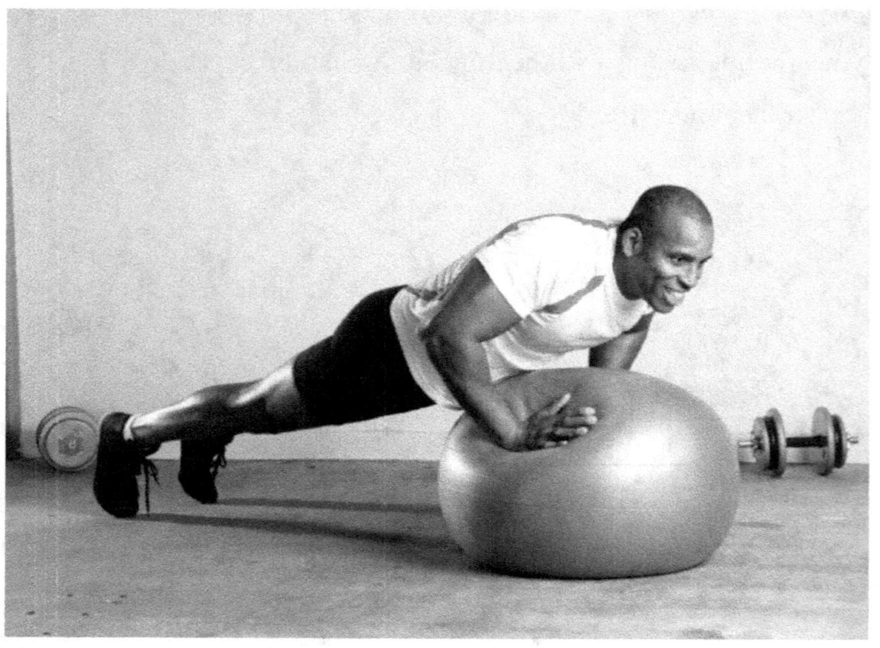

Strength training is important for all ages and fitness levels, as it helps improve muscle tone, build strength and endurance, and improve overall physical health. It can also aid in weight management, improve body composition, and reduce the risk of injury. Additionally, strength training can improve mental health, reduce stress, and improve sleep quality.

When designing a strength training program, it is important to consider individual goals, fitness level, and any existing medical conditions. It is also important to choose exercises that are appropriate for the individual's strength level and to progress gradually as the muscles become stronger. It is also important to ensure that proper form is used and to rest between sets.

Strength training can be done at home or in the gym and can include a variety of exercises, such as weightlifting, bodyweight exercises, plyometrics, and other forms of resistance training. It is important to note that strength training should not be done every day, as this can lead to overtraining and injury. Instead, it is best to incorporate strength training into a weekly routine.

Overall, strength training is an important part of any fitness routine and can help improve overall physical and mental health. It is important to choose exercises that are appropriate for the individual's strength level and to rest between sets. Additionally, strength training should not be done every day, as this can lead to overtraining and injury.

15 Examples of Strength Training Exercises

1. **Squats:** a strength training exercise which involves bending the legs and hips and lowering the body into a squatting position.

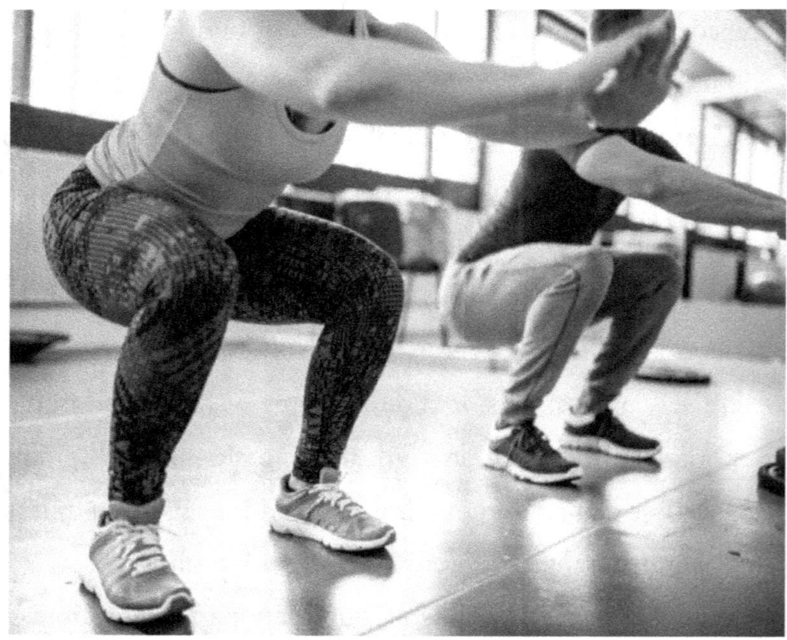

2. **Push-Ups:** A strength training exercise which involves pushing the body up and down off the ground using the arms and chest muscles.

3. **Pull-Ups**: A strength training exercise which involves pulling the body up to a bar suspended above the ground using the arms and back muscles.

4. Lunges: A strength training exercise which involves taking a large step forward and bending the legs and hips to lower the body into a lunge position.

5. Deadlifts: A strength training exercise which involves lifting a weighted barbell from the ground to the hips and then back down again.

6. Bench Press: A strength training exercise which involves pushing a barbell upwards from the chest while lying flat on a bench.

7. Shoulder Press: A strength training exercise which involves pushing a barbell upwards from the shoulder while standing.

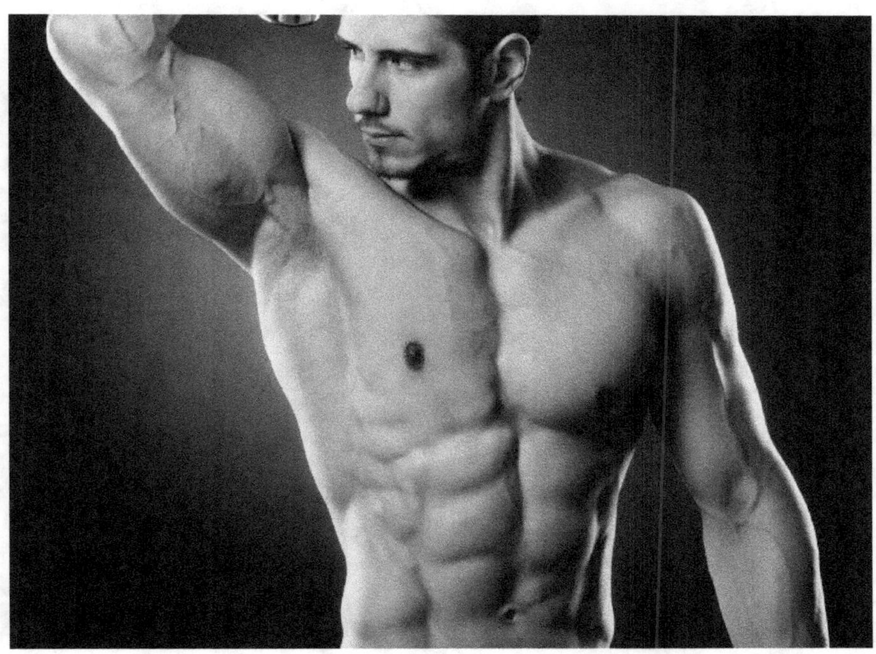

8. Bicep Curls: A strength training exercise which involves curling a weighted barbell or dumbbell upwards from the arm to the shoulder.

9. Tricep Extensions: A strength training exercise which involves extending a weighted barbell or dumbbell downwards from the shoulder to the arm.

10. Lat Pull-Downs: A strength training exercise which involves pulling a weighted barbell downwards from a high place to the chest.

11. Calf Raises: A strength training exercise which involves standing on the balls of the feet and raising the heels off the ground.

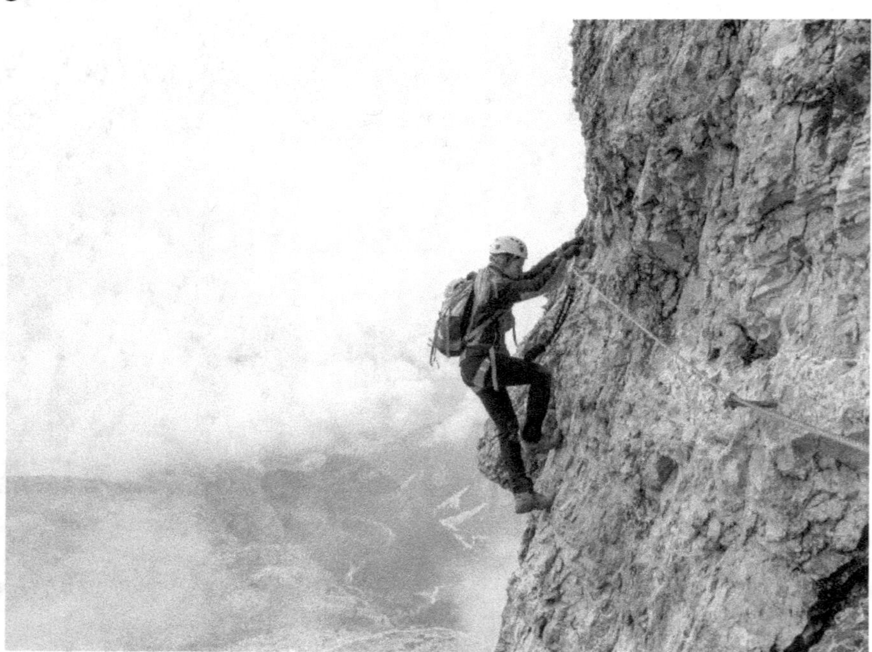

12. Plank: a strength training exercise which involves holding the body in a straight line while balancing on the elbows and toes.

13. Mountain Climbers: a strength training exercise which involves alternating the legs between a running motion while in a plank position.

14. Medicine Ball Slams: a strength training exercise which involves lifting a weighted medicine ball above the head and throwing it into the ground.

15. Russian Twists: a strength training exercise which involves sitting with the legs bent and twisting the torso from side to side while holding a weight.

CARDIOVASCULAR EXERCISE

Any physical activity that raises the heart rate and breathing rate is referred to as cardiovascular exercise. This type of exercise strengthens the heart and lungs and helps to improve overall health. Examples of cardiovascular exercise include walking, running, swimming, cycling, rowing, and aerobics. Regular cardiovascular exercise can help to lower blood pressure and cholesterol levels, reduce stress, and improve endurance. It can also help to reduce the risk of heart disease, stroke, and other medical conditions. To get the most benefit, it is recommended that people engage in at least 30 minutes of moderate-intensity cardiovascular exercise most days of the week.

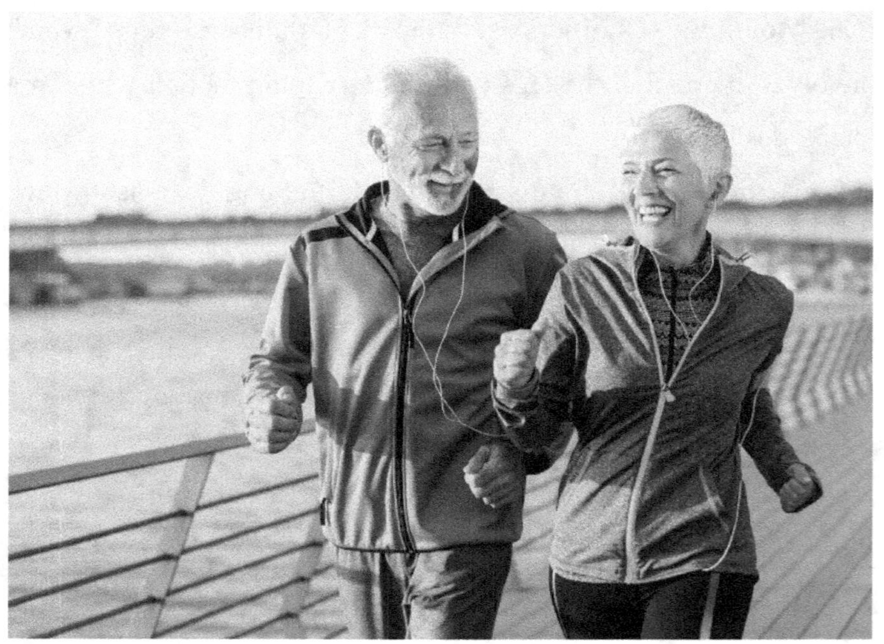

Cardiovascular exercise should be done in a safe and responsible manner. Before beginning any type of physical activity, it is important to consult a doctor to ensure that it is safe for you to do so. When exercising, it is important to warm up, stretch, and cool down properly. Additionally, it is important to drink plenty of water and stay properly hydrated. It is also important to wear comfortable and appropriate clothing and shoes. Finally, it is important to listen to your body and stop exercising if you experience any pain or discomfort.

Exercise for the heart and lungs is crucial to living a healthy lifestyle. By engaging in regular physical activity, you can improve your overall health, reduce stress, and boost your mood.

20 Examples Of Cardiovascular Exercises

1. Running - A great aerobic exercise that involves propelling the body forward by alternating the legs and arms in a rhythmic motion.

2. Jogging - A slower form of running that still involves propelling the body forward by alternating the legs and arms in a rhythmic motion.

3. Swimming - An aerobic exercise that uses all major muscle groups in the body while also providing a low-impact workout.

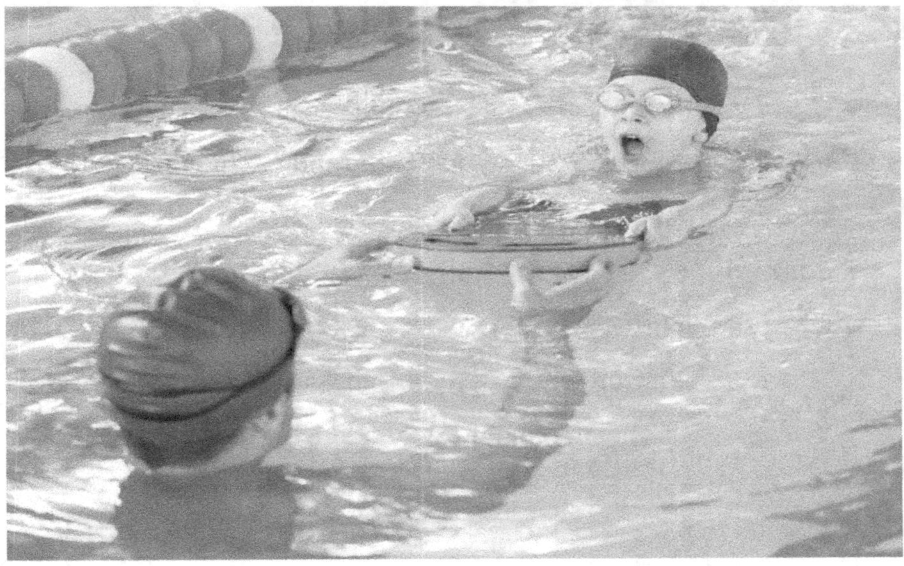

4. Cycling - A great aerobic exercise that uses the muscles in the legs to propel the bike forward.

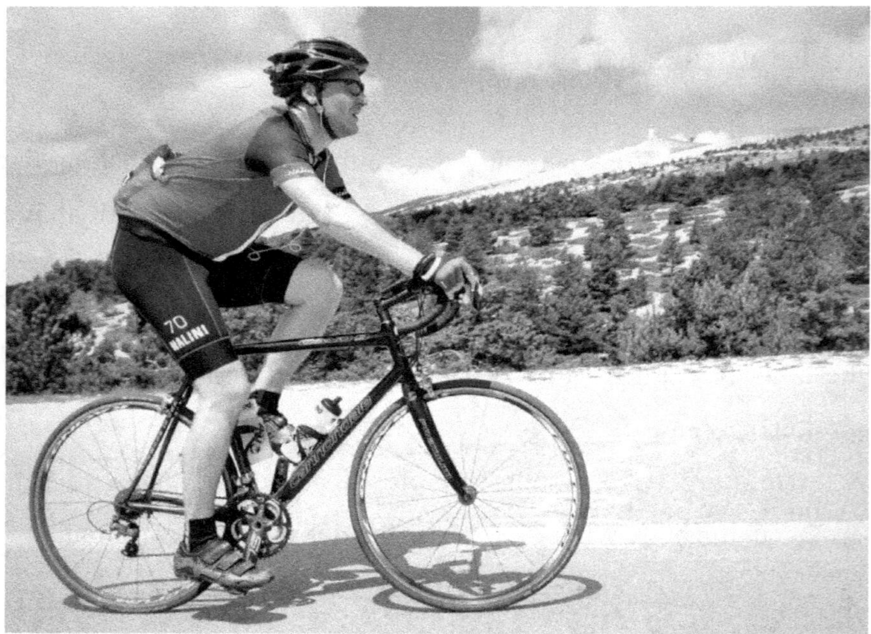

5. Elliptical Trainer – A low-impact exercise machine that allows users to move in a circular motion while providing an aerobic workout.

6. Jump Rope - A great full-body exercise that increases heart rate and helps to improve coordination.

7. Rowing - A great aerobic exercise that uses both the upper and lower body to propel the boat forward.

8. Stair Climbing - A great aerobic exercise that increases heart rate and helps to strengthen the lower body muscles.

9. Burpees - A full-body exercise that involves jumping, squatting, and pushing up in one motion.

10. Skipping - A great aerobic exercise that helps to increase heart rate and strengthen the lower body muscles.

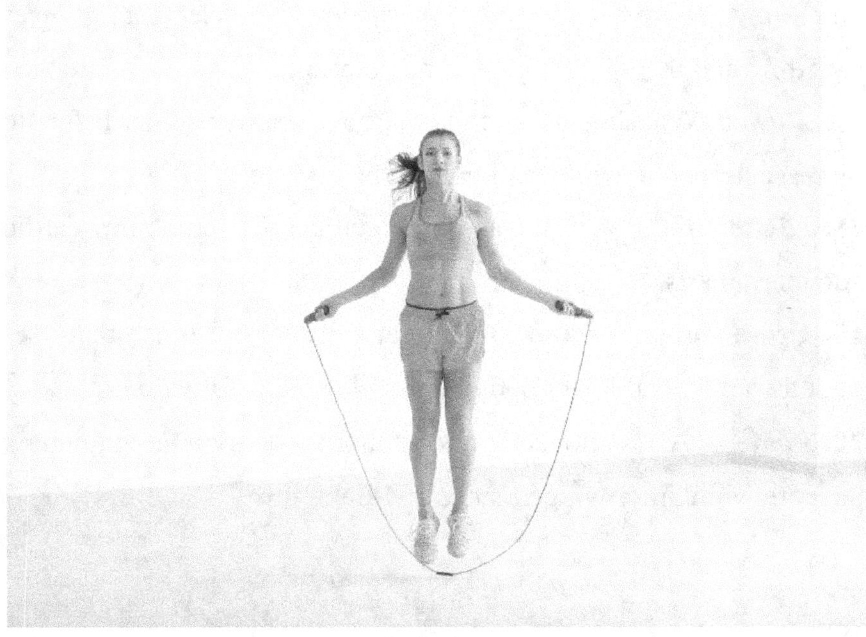

11. Walking - A low-impact exercise that is great for those who are just starting out or are recovering from an injury.

2. Dancing - A great aerobic exercise that combines cardio and fun all in one.

13. Jumping Jacks - A great full-body exercise that uses both the upper and lower body to increase heart rate.

14. High Knees - A great aerobic exercise that helps to increase heart rate and strengthens the lower body muscles.

15. Mountain Climbers - A full-body exercise that involves alternating the legs and arms in an up and down motion.

16. Squat Jumps - A great lower body exercise that involves squatting and then jumping up in one motion.

17. Power Walking - A great aerobic exercise that helps to increase heart rate while walking at a brisk pace.

18. Kickboxing - A great aerobic exercise that combines cardio and martial arts.

19. Cross-Country Skiing - A great full-body exercise that uses both the upper and lower body to propel the skis forward.

20. Pilates - A low-impact exercise that focuses on strengthening the core while improving balance and flexibility.

FLEXIBILITY EXERCISES

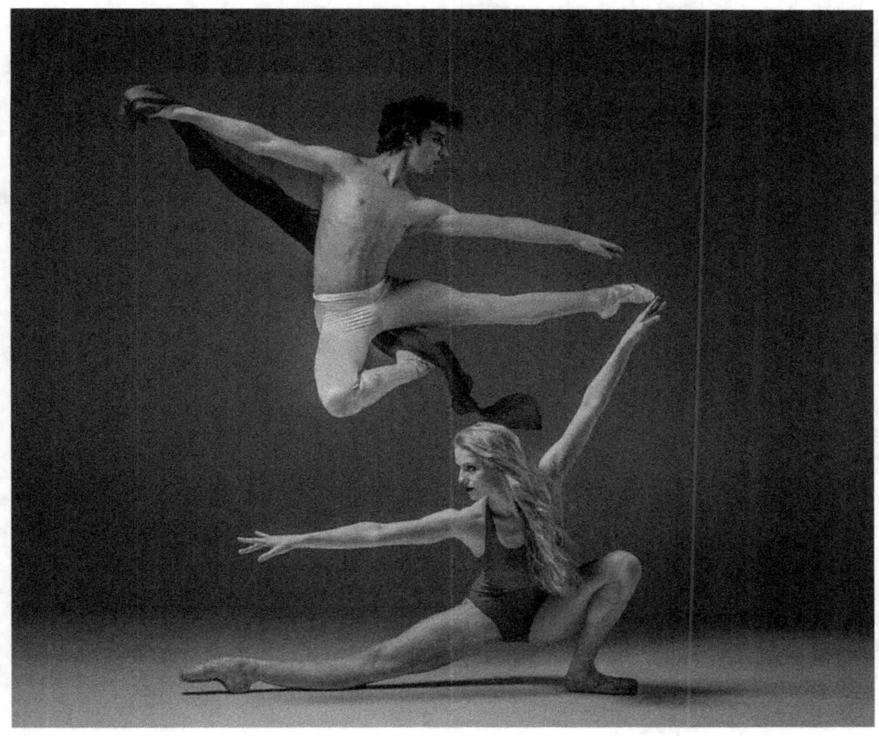

Flexibility exercises are exercises that help improve the range of motion in a joint or muscle group. This can improve your performance in sports or everyday activities and can also help reduce the risk of injuries. Stretching, yoga, Pilates, and foam rolling are a few examples of flexibility exercises.

Stretching is a great way to improve flexibility. It can be done statically, which means holding a stretch for a period of time, or dynamically, which involves moving through the range of motion.

Static stretching is best done after exercise, while dynamic stretching is best done as part of a warm-up.

Yoga is an excellent way to increase flexibility as well as strength and balance. Many poses are designed to stretch and lengthen the muscles and improve the range of motion in the joints.

Pilates is another form of exercise that can help improve flexibility. This type of exercise emphasizes controlled movement and focuses on building core strength.

Foam rolling is a form of self-myofascial release, which is a way to massage and stretch your muscles and fascia. Foam rolling can help improve flexibility, reduce tightness in muscles, and reduce the risk of injury.

By incorporating a variety of flexibility exercises into your fitness routine, you can help improve your overall performance, reduce your risk of injury, and increase your range of motion.

20 Examples Of Flexibility Exercises

1. Cat-Cow Stretch: This stretch helps lengthen the spine and open up the chest and shoulders. It can be done by starting on your hands and knees and then arching your back like a cat, and then lowering your head and chest and rounding the spine like a cow.

2. **Forward Fold:** This is a simple standing hamstring stretch that can be done anywhere. Start standing with your feet hip-width apart and then bend forward from the hips, keeping your knees slightly bent and your back flat as you reach toward your toes.

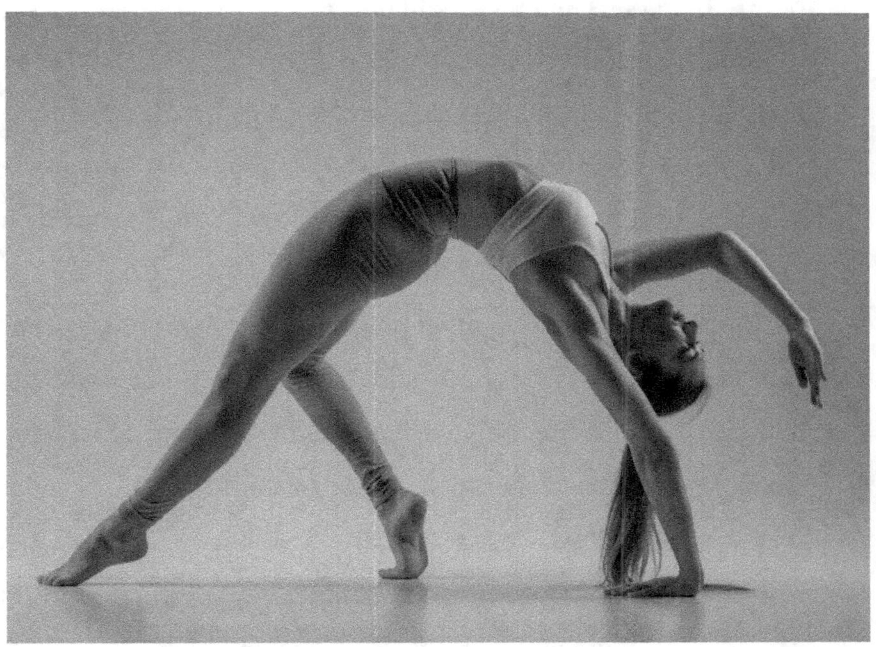

3. **Side Bends**: This stretch helps improve your lateral mobility and flexibility in your shoulders and spine. Start standing with your feet hip-width apart and then reach one arm up and over your head to the other side, bending from the waist and trying to touch the floor.

4. Standing Hamstring Stretch: This stretch targets your hamstrings and helps improve your range of motion in your hips and legs. Start standing with your feet hip-width apart and then bend one knee and reach down to touch your toes. Hold the stretch for 30-60 seconds and then switch legs.

5. Seated Spinal Twist: This is a great way to improve your flexibility and mobility in your spine. Start by sitting on the ground with your legs crossed and then twist your torso to the right, placing your left hand on the floor for support. Hold the stretch for 30-60 seconds and then switch sides.

6. Child's Pose: This is a great pose to help you relax and improve your flexibility in your back and hips. Start by kneeling on the floor and then sit back on your heels and reach your arms forward, letting your head and chest rest on the ground.

7. Downward Dog: This is a great whole-body stretch that helps improve your flexibility in your shoulders, hips, and legs. Start by getting on all fours and then lift your hips up and back, forming an inverted V-shape with your body.

8. Squats: Squats are a great way to improve your overall flexibility and mobility in your lower body. Start by standing with your feet hip-width apart and then lower your body into a squatting position, keeping your chest up and your back straight.

9. Lunges: Lunges are a great way to improve your flexibility and mobility in your lower body. Start by standing with your feet hip-width apart and then step forward with one leg and lower your body into a lunge position, keeping your chest up and your back straight.

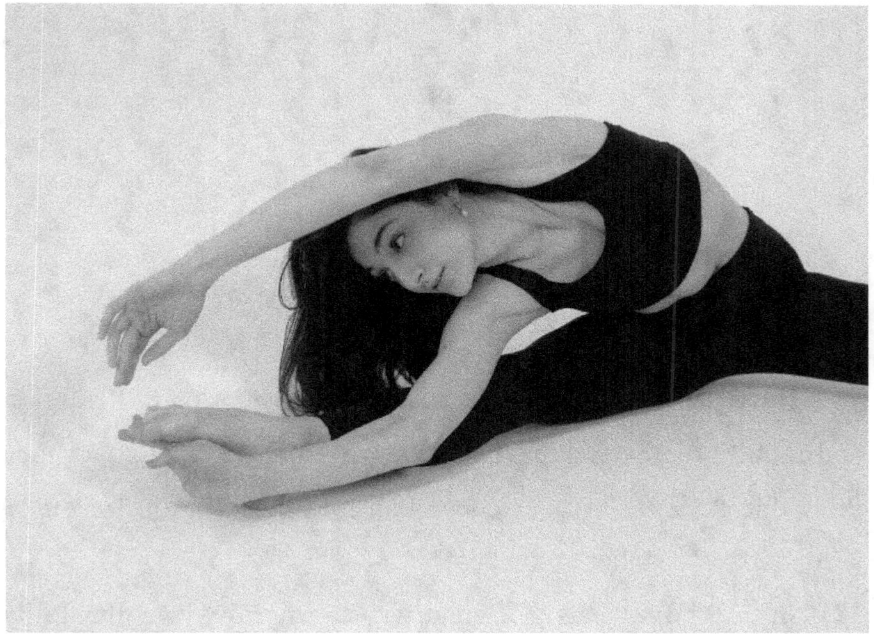

10. Wall Sits: Wall sits are a great way to improve your flexibility and mobility in your lower body. Start by standing with your back against a wall and then slide down until your thighs are parallel to the floor. Hold the position for 30-60 seconds and then stand back up.

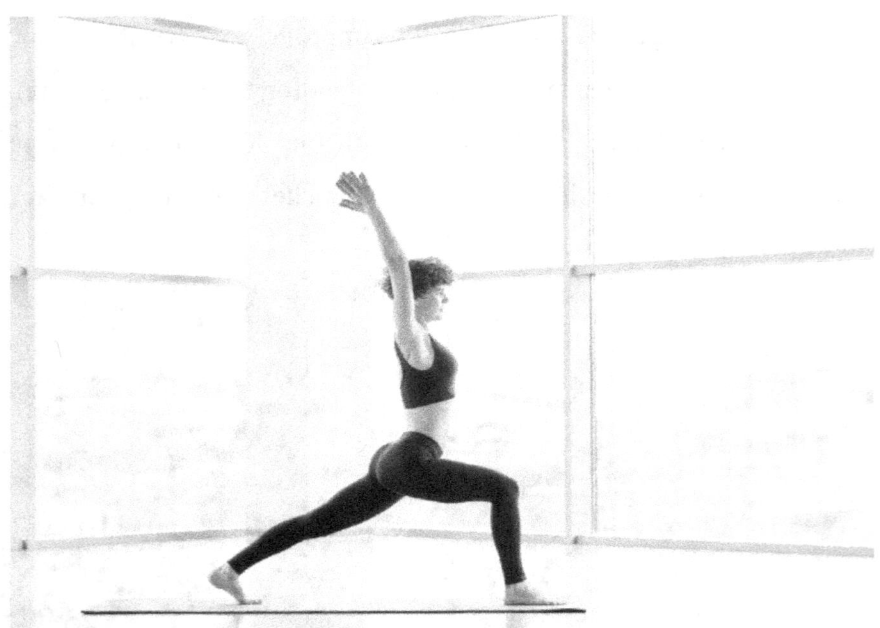

11. Hip Openers: Hip openers are great for improving flexibility and mobility in your hips. Start by lying on your back and then draw one knee up to your chest and hold the position for 30-60 seconds. Switch sides and repeat.

12. Glute Bridge: This is a great way to improve your flexibility and mobility in your lower body. Start by lying on your back and then lift your hips up off the floor, forming a bridge with your body. Hold the position for 30-60 seconds and then lower your hips back to the floor.

13. Trunk Rotations: This is a great way to improve your flexibility and mobility in your torso. Start by lying on your back and then rotate your torso from side to side, keeping your arms outstretched and your feet on the ground.

14. Shoulder Rolls: Shoulder rolls are a great way to improve your flexibility and mobility in your shoulders. Start by standing with your feet hip-width apart and then roll your shoulders back and forth, keeping your arms relaxed at your sides.

15. Neck Stretches: Neck stretches are a great way to improve your flexibility and mobility in your neck. Start by standing with your feet hip-width apart and then gently tilt your head to the left, right, and then back. Hold each position for 30-60 seconds.

16. Push-Ups: Push-ups are a great way to improve your overall strength and flexibility. Start by getting into a plank position and then lower your body down until your chest touches the ground. Push back up and repeat.

17. Plank: Planks are a great way to improve your overall strength and flexibility. Start by getting into a push-up position and then hold your body in a straight line, making sure your hips do not sag. Hold the position for 30-60 seconds and then relax.

18. Single-Leg Balance: This is a great way to improve your overall balance and flexibility. Start by standing on one foot and then lift the other foot off the ground. Hold the position for 30-60 seconds and then switch sides.

19. Knee to Chest: This is a great way to improve your flexibility in your lower back. Start by lying on your back and then draw one knee up to your chest and hold the position for 30-60 seconds. Switch sides and repeat.

20. Ankle Circles: This is a great way to improve your flexibility in your ankles. Start by standing with your feet hip-width apart and then draw circles with your ankles in one direction for 30-60 seconds and then switch directions.

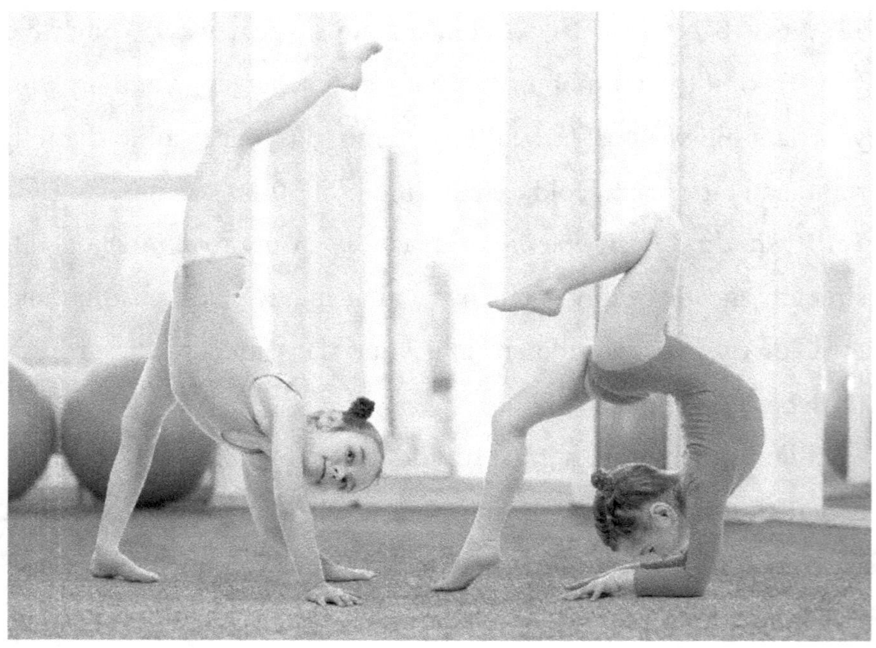

CHAPTER THREE

MENTAL HEALTH FOR LONGEVITY

Mental health is an integral part of our overall well-being and is essential for longevity. Mental health affects our physical health, our ability to manage stress, our relationships, and our overall quality of life. As such, it is important to take steps to maintain good mental health.

One of the most important things to do for your mental health is to practice self-care. This include getting enough rest, eating well, working out frequently, and setting aside time for yourself. Taking care of your mental health also means recognizing and managing any stress, anxiety, depression, or other mental health issues that you may be experiencing.

Also, it's essential that you maintain an optimistic mindset. Practicing gratitude and looking for the good in every situation can help to boost both your physical and mental health. Connecting with people, especially those you care about, is also important for your mental health. Making time for yourself and engaging in activities that bring you joy, such as hobbies or creative pursuits, can help to improve your mental health.

It is important to seek professional help if you are struggling with mental health issues. Mental health professionals can provide guidance, support, and treatment to help you better manage your mental health and improve your quality of life.

Maintaining good mental health is essential for longevity. By taking steps to prioritize your mental health, you can help to ensure that you are living your life to the fullest.

STRESS MANAGEMENT

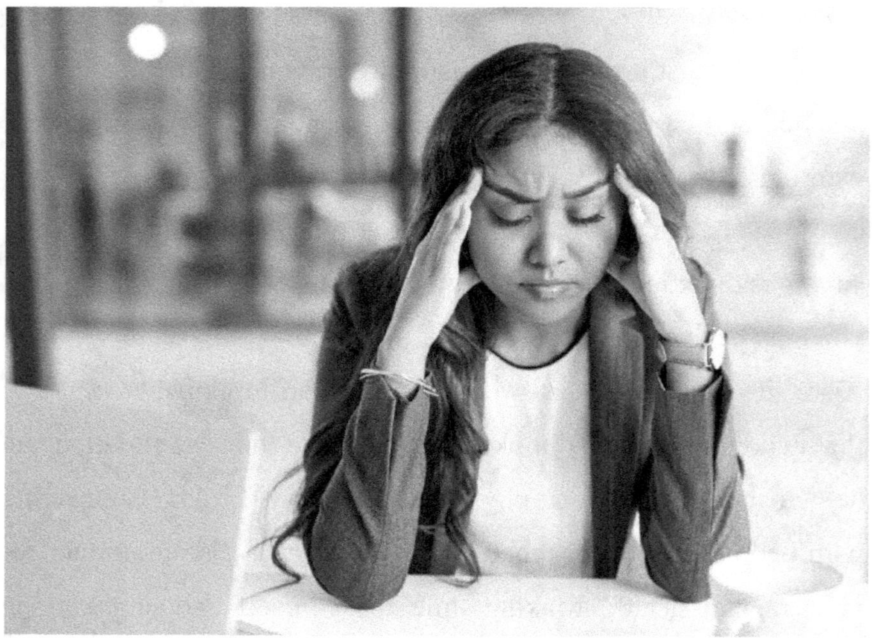

Stress is an unavoidable part of life, but it doesn't have to be debilitating. With the right tools and techniques, you can learn how to manage stress and make it work for you.

The first step to stress management is to identify the sources of stress in your life. Make a list of everything causing you worry and anxiety, from work deadlines to financial worries. Once you've identified the sources of your stress, you can begin to take steps to manage it.

Take some time each day to relax and reset your mind. This could be as simple as taking a few minutes to meditate or journaling your thoughts. Taking time to relax will help you reduce stress and find clarity.

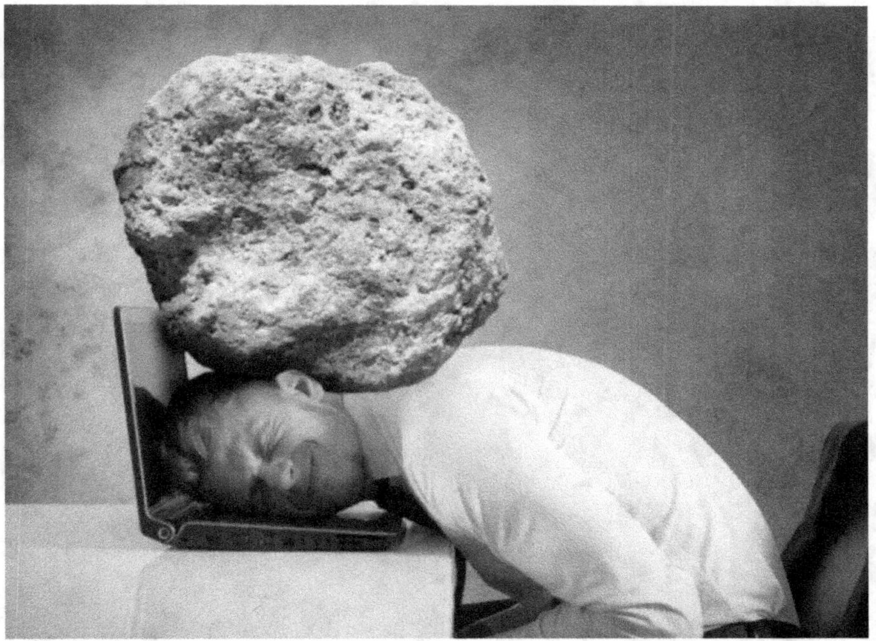

Exercising is another great way to manage stress. Exercise releases endorphins which can lift your mood and help you release tension. A small amount of exercise each day can have a significant impact.

Plan time specifically for your favorite activities. Whether it's reading, listening to music, or spending time with friends, taking time for yourself can help you manage stress and give you a sense of purpose.

Also, make sure to get adequate sleep. Insufficient sleep can make stress worse and make it more difficult to handle. Try to sleep for seven to eight hours per night. Stress management is all about learning how to cope with stress in a healthy way. With practice, you can learn how to use stress to your advantage and make it a positive force in your life.

15 Ways Of Managing Stress

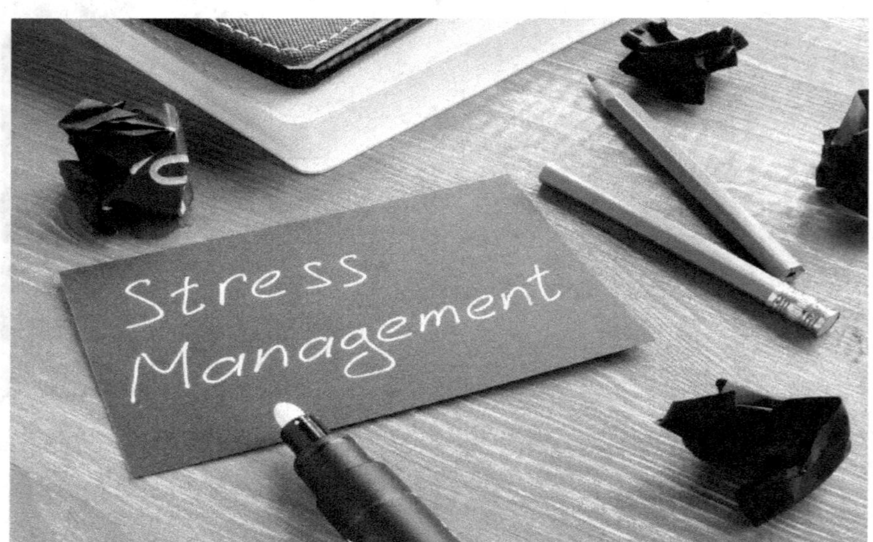

1. Exercise: Regular exercise is a great way to reduce stress levels. Exercise releases endorphins which can help to reduce stress and make you feel better overall.

2. Eat healthy: Eating a balanced diet can help to reduce stress levels. Eating foods that are high in vitamins and minerals can help to provide the body with the nutrition it needs to handle stress better.

3. Get enough sleep: Sleep is essential for reducing stress and helping the body to recover from stressful situations.

4. Laugh: Laughter can be an effective way to reduce stress levels, as it helps to relax the body and mind.

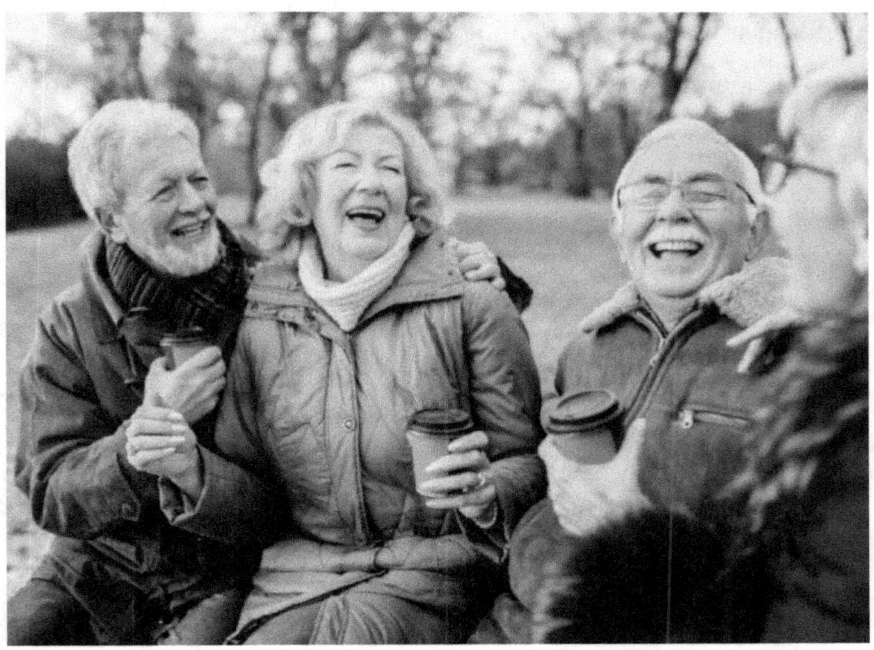

5. Connect with people: Connecting with friends and family is a great way to reduce stress. Talking to people who understand you and can offer support can help to reduce stress levels.

6. Take breaks: Taking regular breaks throughout the day can help to reduce stress levels.

7. Meditate: Meditation is a great way to reduce stress and help the mind to relax.

8. Practice deep breathing: Deep breathing can help to reduce stress levels. Taking slow, deep breaths can help to relax the body and mind.

9. Avoid caffeine and alcohol: Caffeine and alcohol can both increase stress levels. Avoiding them can help to reduce stress.

10. Use aromatherapy: Aromatherapy can be an effective way to reduce stress. Essential oils such as lavender, lemon, and chamomile can help to relax the body and mind.

11. Listen to music: Listening to calming music can help to reduce stress levels and make you feel more relaxed.

12. Practice yoga: Yoga is a great way to reduce stress levels. It can help to relax the body and mind and reduce stress.

13. Take a walk: Taking a walk can be a great way to reduce stress levels. The fresh air and exercise can help to relax the body and mind.

14. Read a book: Reading can be a great way to reduce stress levels. It can help to take your mind off of whatever is causing the stress and help you to relax.

15. Journal: Writing down your thoughts and feelings can be a great way to reduce stress. It can help to get your feelings out and give you a better perspective on the situation.

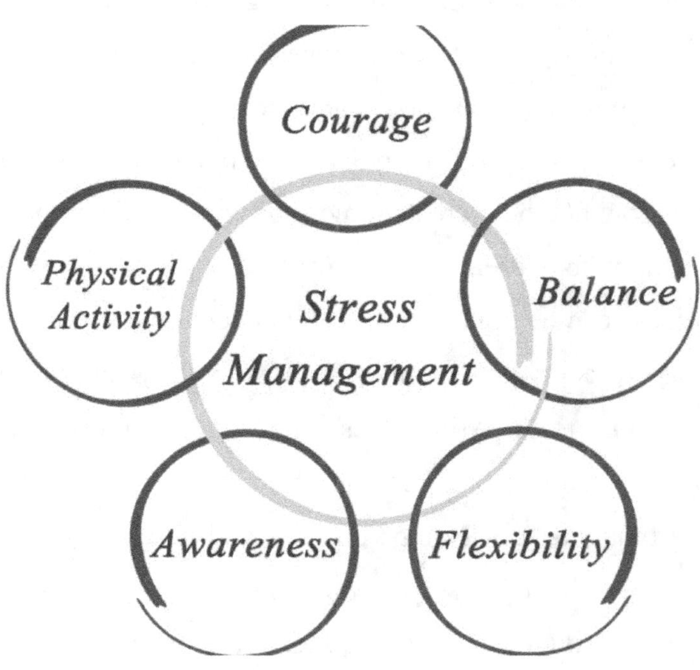

MINDFULNESS

Mindfulness is a psychological practice in which an individual focuses on the present moment and their inner experience with an attitude of openness, curiosity, and non-judgment. It is a way to pay attention to one's thoughts, feelings, and bodily sensations with a spirit of acceptance and kindness. Mindfulness has its roots in Buddhist meditation practices and is often considered a type of meditation. When practiced regularly, it can reduce stress, improve concentration, and help create a more balanced and compassionate relationship with oneself and the world.

Mindfulness can be practiced in many different ways, from formal meditation to everyday activities such as eating, walking, or even brushing your teeth. Mindfulness meditation typically involves sitting in a comfortable position, focusing on the breath, and allowing thoughts and feelings to come and go without judgment. It can also involve body scans, where the individual pays attention to different parts of the body and mentally notices any sensations that may be present.

Mindfulness can be beneficial for both physical and mental health. It can help people become more aware of their thoughts and emotions, allowing them to develop better self-awareness, self-regulation, and self-compassion. In addition, mindfulness can help reduce stress, improve concentration, and increase positive emotions. Furthermore, it can help individuals become more compassionate and connected to others, leading to deeper and more Mindfulness is a powerful tool that can be used to develop greater psychological well-being and improve overall mental health. It is a practice that can be integrated into any lifestyle and is suitable for people of all ages and backgrounds.

MENTAL STIMULATION

Mental stimulation is thought to be an important part of maintaining a healthy, active lifestyle and can help to increase longevity. Studies have shown that people who engage in mentally stimulating activities on a regular basis have a lower risk of developing age-related diseases and memory loss.

Mental stimulation can help to keep the brain active and healthy, leading to better overall physical and mental health. It can also help to delay the onset of age-related declines in cognitive function. Examples of mentally stimulating activities include reading, playing board games, puzzles, and engaging in conversations with friends.

The effects of mental stimulation can help to increase longevity and quality of life. Studies have shown that people who engage in mental activities on a regular basis have a lower risk of developing

Alzheimer's disease and other forms of dementia. Mental stimulation can also help to reduce stress and anxiety levels, which can lead to better sleep and overall better health.

Mental stimulation can also help to keep the mind sharp and alert. By engaging in mentally stimulating activities, individuals can help to improve their memory, focus, and problem-solving ability. This can lead to increased productivity and a longer, healthier life. Overall, mental stimulation is an important part of maintaining a healthy, active lifestyle and can help to increase longevity. Engaging in mentally stimulating activities on a regular basis can help to reduce the risk of age-related diseases, improve cognitive function, reduce stress, and improve overall health and wellbeing.

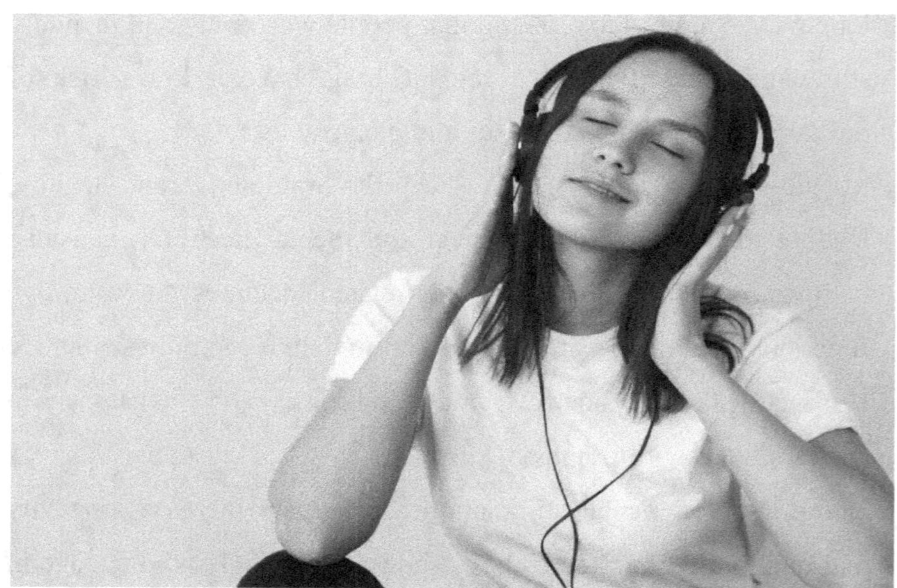

20 Mental Stimulation Activities

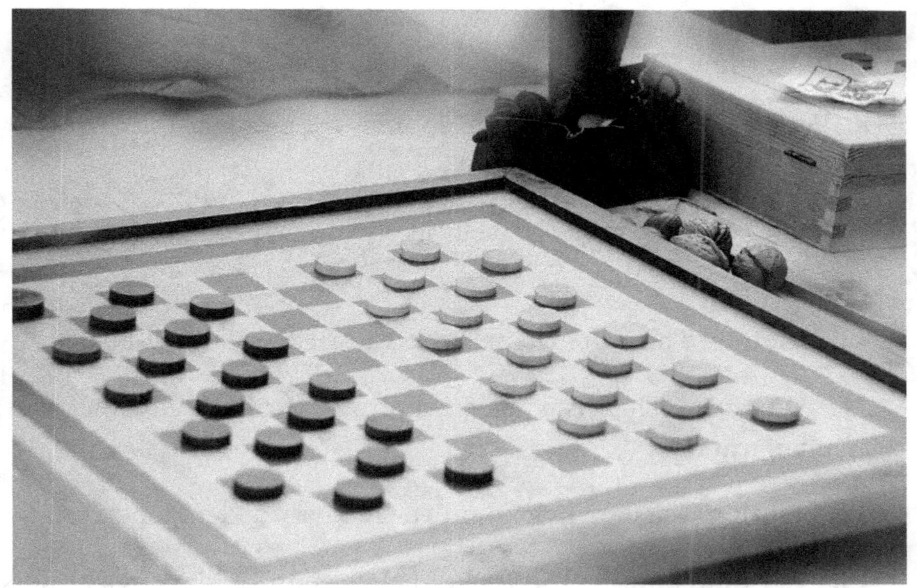

1. Crossword puzzles: These can help improve memory and problem-solving skills.

2. Brain teasers: These can help improve problem-solving skills and mental agility.

3. Word searches: These can help improve memory and visual recognition skills.

4. Sudoku: This requires logic and reasoning skills, and helps improve them.

5. Chess: This requires concentration, problem-solving, and strategy.

6. Trivia games: These can help improve knowledge and mental agility.

7. Memory games: These can help improve memory, concentration, and recall.

8. Jigsaw puzzles: These can help improve problem-solving skills and spatial reasoning.

9. Card games: These can help improve concentration, memory, and strategy.

10. Reading: This can help improve knowledge and vocabulary.

11. Writing: This can help improve creative thinking and communication.

12. Painting: This can help improve creativity and motor skills.

13. Scrapbooking: This can help improve creativity and organization.

14. Listening to music: This can help improve relaxation and focus.

15. Yoga: This can help improve relaxation and physical fitness.

16. Gardening: This can help improve relaxation and motor skills.

17. Cooking: This can help improve problem-solving and creativity.

18. Taking photographs: This can help improve creativity and visual recognition.

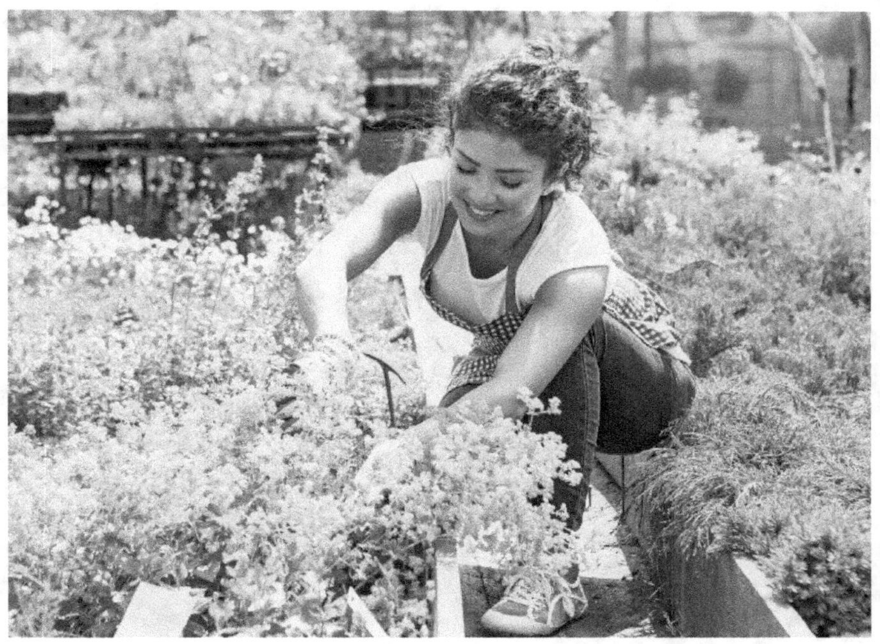

19. Taking classes: This can help improve knowledge and learning skills.

20. Volunteering: This can help improve social skills and empathy.

CHAPTER FOUR

MANAGING CHRONIC ILLNESSES

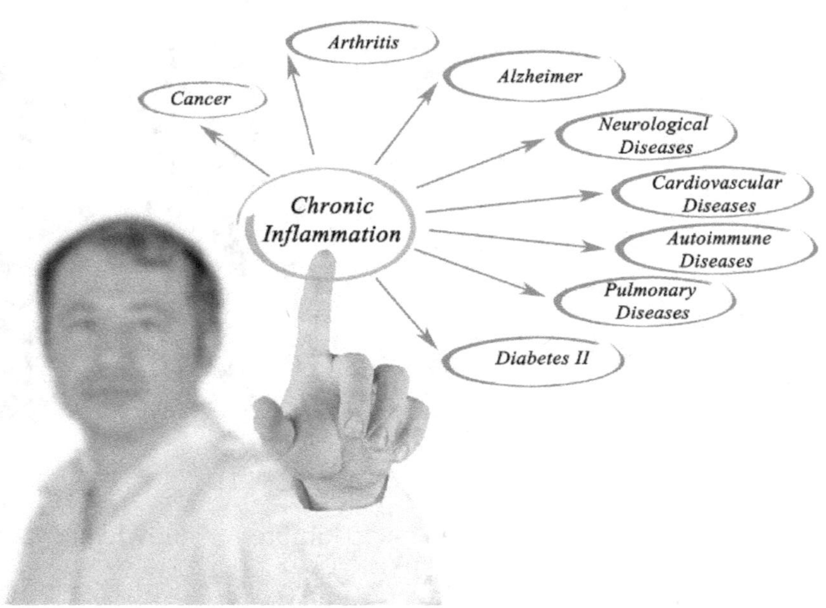

Managing chronic illnesses can be a daunting task for those affected by them. It is important to understand the importance of self-care and how it can help reduce the severity of symptoms and improve quality of life.

The most important step in managing chronic illnesses is to stay informed. It is important to learn about the illness, its treatments, and the risks associated with it. This can help individuals understand their condition better and make informed decisions about their care. It is also essential to stay in contact with healthcare providers to ensure that any changes in treatment are properly monitored.

In addition to staying informed, developing a healthy lifestyle is essential for managing chronic illnesses. This includes exercising regularly, eating a balanced diet, and avoiding unhealthy activities such as smoking and excessive drinking. Regular physical activity can help increase energy levels and reduce stress, while eating a balanced diet can benefit overall health.

It is also important to practice self-care when managing chronic illnesses. This includes finding the right balance between rest and activity, following a regular sleep schedule, and taking time to relax and unwind. Additionally, it is important to recognize and accept any limitations that come with a chronic illness and to ensure that any necessary accommodations are made.

It is important to stay connected with a support network. This can include family, friends, and healthcare providers. These individuals can provide emotional support, guidance, and practical help in managing chronic illnesses.

Managing chronic illnesses can be a difficult and challenging process. However, with the right knowledge and support, it is possible to maintain a good quality of life.

By understanding the importance of staying informed, developing a healthy lifestyle, practicing self-care, and connecting with a support network, individuals can take the steps necessary to manage their chronic illnesses and lead a fulfilling life.

DIABETES

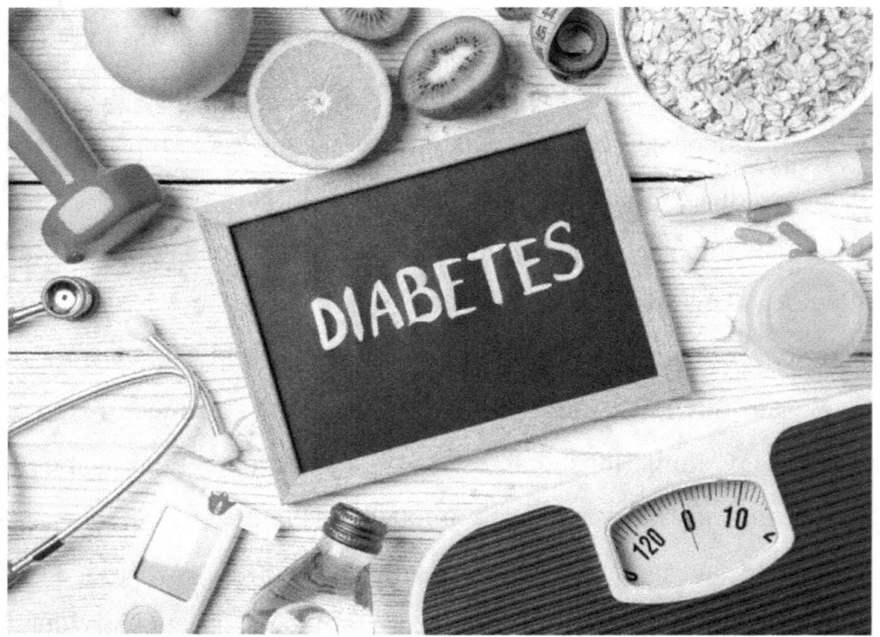

Diabetes is a chronic, metabolic disease which is characterized by high blood sugar levels (hyperglycemia) over a prolonged period of time. It is a condition in which the body either does not produce enough insulin, or cannot effectively use the insulin it produces, resulting in an inability to adequately regulate sugar levels. Diabetes affects millions of people worldwide and is one of the leading causes of death and disability.

The two main types of diabetes are type 1 and type 2. Type 1 diabetes is caused by an autoimmune response which destroys the insulin-producing cells in the pancreas, thus requiring the patient to take regular injections of insulin. Type 2 diabetes, however, is usually caused by lifestyle factors such as poor diet, physical inactivity, and obesity. It is more common than type 1 diabetes, accounting for 90-95% of all cases.

The most common symptoms of diabetes include frequent urination, excessive thirst, weight loss, fatigue, and blurred vision. If left untreated, diabetes can lead to serious complications such as heart disease, stroke, kidney failure, blindness, and nerve damage.

The good news is that diabetes can be managed and even prevented with lifestyle changes such as eating a healthy diet, exercising regularly, and maintaining a healthy weight. Eating a balanced diet that is low in saturated fats and high in fiber is important, as is increasing physical activity. Regular exercise helps to control blood sugar levels and can also reduce the risk of developing type 2 diabetes.

In addition to lifestyle changes, medications such as insulin, oral medications, and injectable medications can be used to control blood sugar levels. It is important to speak to a doctor about the best course of treatment for diabetes, as each person's condition is different.

Diabetes is a serious condition, but with proper management and lifestyle changes, it can be managed and even prevented. By eating a healthy diet, exercising regularly, and maintaining a healthy weight, people can reduce their risk of developing diabetes and reduce their symptoms if they already have it. It is important to speak to a doctor about the best course of treatment for diabetes as each person's condition is different. With the right treatment plan, diabetes can be managed and even prevented.

Diabetes can have a significant impact on longevity. People with diabetes have higher rates of mortality than those without the condition. This is especially true if diabetes is not properly managed. People with diabetes are more likely to suffer from a variety of chronic illnesses, such as heart disease, stroke, kidney failure, and blindness. These conditions often lead to premature death and reduced life expectancy. In addition, uncontrolled diabetes can cause nerve and blood vessel damage, which can lead to a wide range of complications, including poor circulation, foot ulcers, and amputations. All of these issues can affect a person's ability to lead a healthy and productive life and ultimately limit their lifespan. It is important to work with a doctor to ensure that diabetes is properly managed in order to reduce the risk of complications and extend longevity.

10 Ways To Prevent Diabetes

1. Exercise regularly: Regular physical activity can help you maintain a healthy weight and lower your risk for diabetes.

2. Eat a healthy diet: Choose foods that are low in saturated fat and added sugars and high in fiber.

3. Maintain a healthy weight: Being overweight increases your risk for developing diabetes.

4. Monitor your blood sugar: Regularly monitor your blood sugar levels and keep them in a healthy range.

5. Don't smoke: Smoking increases your risk of developing diabetes.

6. Get enough sleep: Lack of sleep can increase your risk of developing diabetes.

7. Limit alcohol consumption: Drinking too much alcohol can increase your risk of developing diabetes.

8. Take your medications as prescribed: If you are taking medications to control your blood sugar, follow your doctor's instructions.

9. Get regular check-ups: Regular check-ups with your doctor can help you monitor your blood sugar levels.

10. Monitor your blood pressure: High blood pressure increases your risk of developing diabetes.

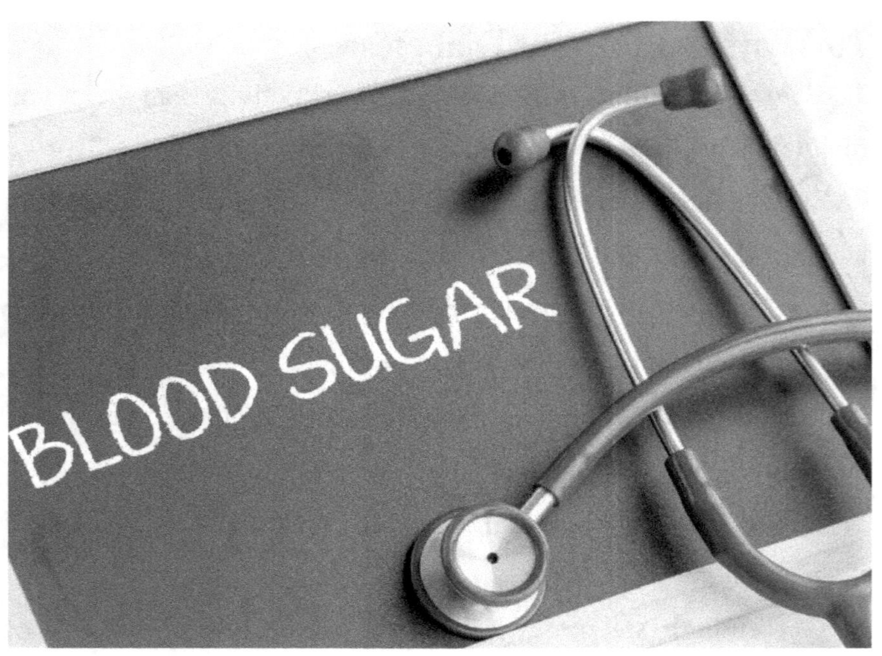

HIGH BLOOD PRESSURE

High blood pressure (hypertension) is a serious health condition that can have life-threatening consequences. It is caused by elevated pressure in the arteries that carry blood from the heart to the rest of the body. It can cause heart disease, strokes, and other significant health issues if left untreated.

High blood pressure is classified into two categories; primary or essential hypertension, and secondary hypertension. Primary hypertension is the most common type and is caused by a combination of lifestyle, environmental, and genetic factors. Secondary hypertension is associated with an underlying medical condition, such as kidney disease or an endocrine disorder.

The primary risk factors for hypertension include obesity, poor diet, lack of physical activity, smoking, and excessive alcohol consumption. High levels of stress and anxiety can also contribute to high blood pressure. Even though there is no single known cause of hypertension, it is important to take steps to reduce the risk.

Making lifestyle changes is the first step in managing high blood pressure. Eating a healthy diet with lots of fruits, vegetables, and whole grains can help reduce blood pressure. Exercise is also important, as it helps to reduce stress levels and increase blood flow. Keeping a healthy weight and quitting smoking can also help to improve blood pressure.

There are also medications available to assist control high blood pressure. These medications work by either blocking the action of certain hormones that can raise blood pressure, or by dilating the vessels that carry blood, allowing it to flow more freely.

High blood pressure is a serious health condition that can have serious consequences. It is important to take steps to reduce the risk of hypertension, including making lifestyle changes and taking medications as prescribed. Taking these steps can help to reduce the risk of serious health complications associated with high blood pressure.

To keep an eye on blood pressure, it's also critical to visit the doctor frequently. Regular check-ups can help identify any changes in blood pressure that need to be addressed. By making lifestyle changes, taking medications as prescribed, and seeing a doctor regularly, people can help reduce the risks associated with high blood pressure and live a full and healthy life.

15 Ways To Prevent High Blood Pressure

1. Maintain a healthy weight. Being overweight or obese increases your risk of developing high blood pressure.

2. Exercise regularly. Regular physical activity helps you maintain a healthy weight and can lower your blood pressure.

3. Eat a healthy diet. Eating a diet rich in fruits, vegetables, whole grains and low-fat dairy products can help lower your blood pressure.

4. Reduce sodium in your diet. A diet high in sodium can lead to higher blood pressure.

5. Limit alcohol consumption. Drinking too much alcohol can raise your blood pressure.

6. Don't smoke. Smoking increases your risk of developing high blood pressure.

7. Reduce stress. Stress can cause your blood pressure to rise.

8. Monitor your blood pressure. Checking your blood pressure regularly can help you stay aware of your risk for high blood pressure.

9. Take medications as prescribed. If your doctor has prescribed medication to lower your blood pressure, take it as directed.

10. Get enough sleep. Not getting enough sleep can increase your risk of developing high blood pressure.

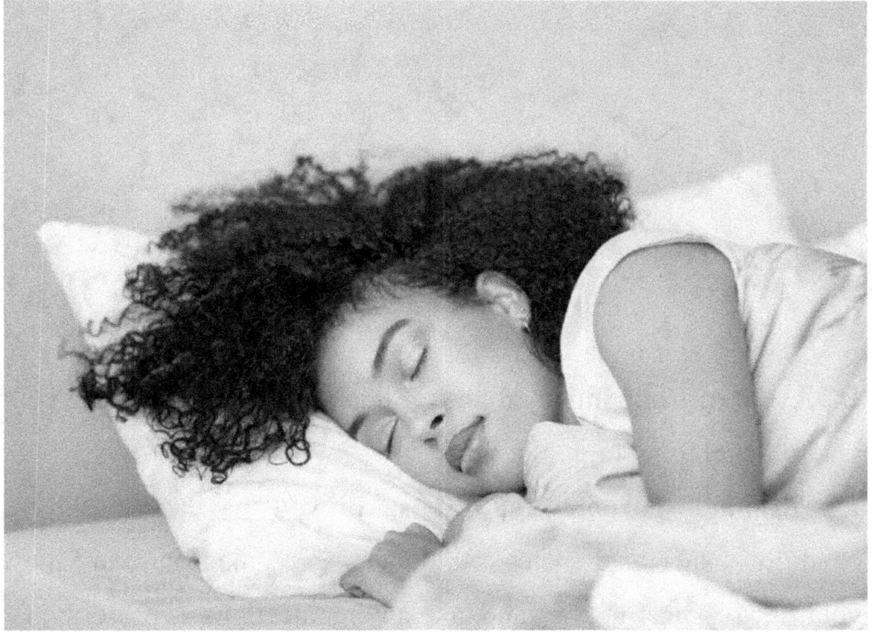

11. Limit caffeine. Too much caffeine can cause your blood pressure to rise.

12. Eat potassium-rich foods. Potassium-rich foods can help lower your blood pressure.

13. Avoid processed and fried foods. These types of foods can raise your blood pressure.

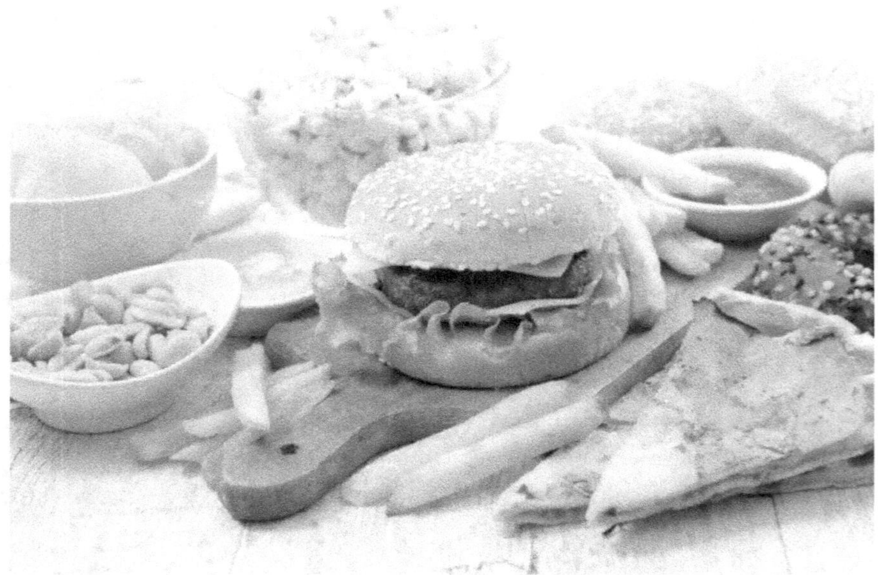

14. Avoid or limit sugary drinks. Sugary drinks can increase your risk of developing high blood pressure.

15. Manage chronic conditions. If you have any chronic conditions, such as diabetes or kidney disease, make sure to follow your doctor's instructions and take any medications as prescribed.

ARTHRITIS

Millions of individuals worldwide suffer from the chronic illness of arthritis. It is a complex disorder that causes inflammation and pain in the joints, as well as damage to the tissue and cartilage surrounding the joints. It can be caused by a variety of factors, including genetics, age, lifestyle, and injury.

The most common type of arthritis is osteoarthritis, which is caused by wear and tear on the cartilage between the bones in the joints. Although it can affect anyone at any age, it is more prevalent among older folks. Symptoms of osteoarthritis include stiffness, pain, and swelling in the joints. The pain may be worse after activity, but can also become worse over time.

Rheumatoid arthritis is another form of arthritis that is caused by an autoimmune disorder. This type of arthritis is more common in women, and can affect any age group. Stiffness, discomfort, and swelling in the joints are signs of osteoarthritis. Moreover, it may result in fever and exhaustion.

Gout is another form of arthritis, and is caused by an accumulation of uric acid crystals in the joints. Men and people over the age of 40 are more likely to experience it. Symptoms of gout include intense pain, swelling, and redness in the joints.

The kind and severity of the arthritis condition will determine how it is treated. Pain and inflammation are frequently treated with non-steroidal anti-inflammatory medications (NSAIDs). Physical therapy and exercise can also help to reduce pain and improve joint mobility. In some cases, surgery may be needed to repair damaged joints or to replace them with artificial ones.

No matter the type of arthritis, the key to managing the condition is to stay active and maintain a healthy lifestyle. Eating a healthy diet, exercising regularly, and getting adequate rest can help to reduce pain and inflammation. It is also important to talk to your doctor about any medication you are taking to make sure it is not making the condition worse.

Arthritis can be a difficult and painful condition to live with, but there are ways to manage it and maintain a good quality of life. The appropriate course of action for your specific circumstance should be discussed with your doctor. With proper treatment and lifestyle changes, you can reduce your pain and improve your overall health.

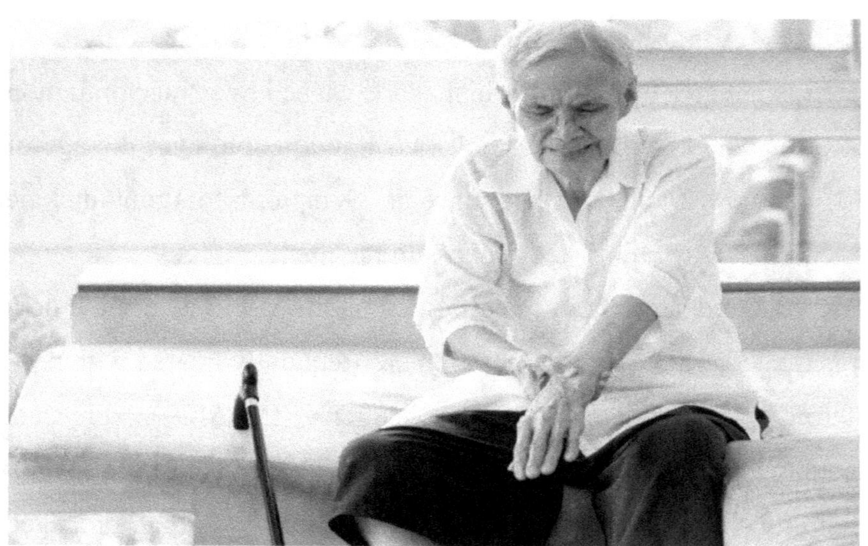

15 Ways To Prevent Arthritis

1. Exercise Regularly: Exercise helps keep joints flexible, strengthens muscles, and improves balance, coordination, and posture.

2. Maintain a Healthy Weight: Excess weight puts extra strain on joints, particularly the hips and knees.

3. Eat a Healthy Diet: Eating a diet rich in fruits, vegetables, and whole grains, and low in processed foods, saturated fat, and sugar helps reduce inflammation in the body.

4. Avoid Injury: Take precautions to avoid falls and other injuries that could lead to joint damage.

5. Avoid Repetitive Movements: Repetitive movements, such as typing or lifting, can put strain on the joints and lead to arthritis.

6. Use Heat and Cold Therapy: Applying heat or cold to the affected joint can help relieve pain and stiffness.

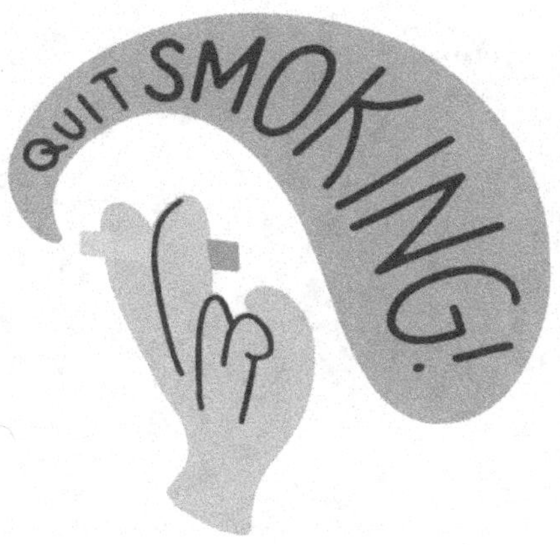

7. Quit Smoking: Smoking increases the risk of developing arthritis, particularly rheumatoid arthritis.

8. Avoid Overusing Joints: Take regular breaks from activities that require repetitive motions and allow your joints to rest.

9. Take Supplements: Omega-3 fatty acids, glucosamine, and chondroitin may help reduce joint pain.

10. Use Assistive Devices: Assistive devices, such as canes and walkers, can help decrease the strain on joints.

11. Try Acupuncture: Acupuncture can help reduce joint pain and inflammation.

12. Take Medication: Nonsteroidal anti-inflammatory drugs (NSAIDs) can help reduce inflammation and pain.

13. Practice Yoga: Regularly practicing yoga can increase flexibility, reduce pain, and improve joint function.

14. Get Enough Sleep: Getting enough sleep helps the body to repair itself, which can help reduce pain and inflammation.

15. Stay Hydrated: Drinking plenty of water can help keep joints lubricated and reduce joint pain.

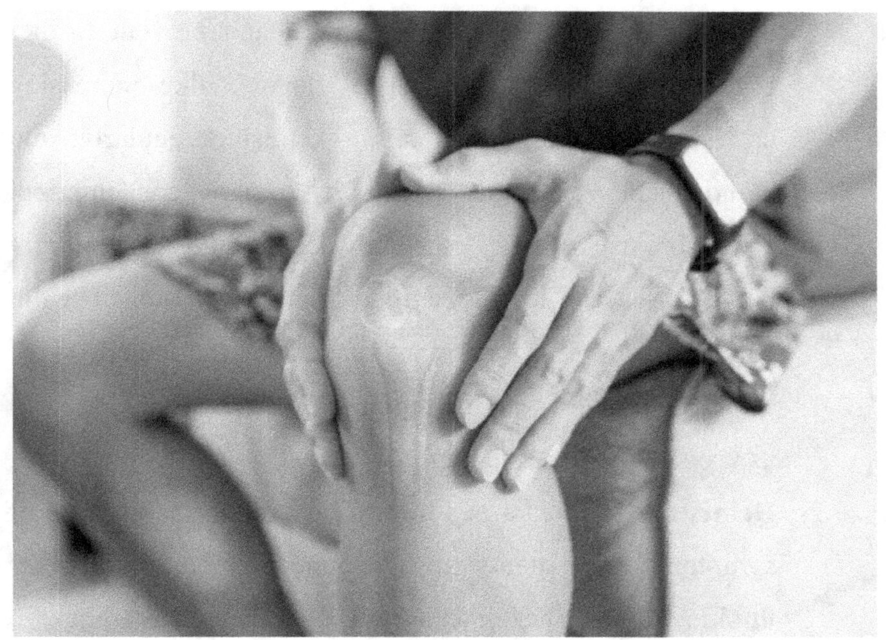

OTHER SICKNESSES ASSOCIATED WITH OLD AGE

1. **Osteoporosis:** Osteoporosis is a condition that affects elderly people and causes bones to become brittle and weak. It is usually caused by a lack of calcium and vitamin D in the diet, as well as hormonal changes that occur with age. As bones become weaker, they can easily break or fracture from a fall or injury. There are medications

available to help treat the condition and prevent further bone loss, as well as lifestyle changes like increasing calcium and vitamin D intake, exercising regularly, and avoiding smoking and excessive alcohol consumption. Osteoporosis can be especially concerning for elderly people, as it can lead to serious fractures and other health complications. It is important for elderly individuals to be aware of the signs and symptoms of osteoporosis, as well as ways to prevent and treat it.

2. **Dementia**: Dementia is a term used to describe a group of symptoms associated with a decline in memory or other thinking skills that interfere with a person's ability to perform everyday activities. It is most commonly seen in elderly people, although it can affect people of any age. Dementia is caused by physical changes in the brain, which can be due to a variety of conditions, such as Alzheimer's disease, stroke, Parkinson's disease, and Huntington's disease. Symptoms of dementia can include memory loss, difficulty with communication, confusion, difficulty with problem solving, difficulty with planning, and changes in mood and behavior. The exact cause of dementia is not known, but age, lifestyle, and genetics can be contributing factors. Treatments for dementia vary depending on the underlying cause, but may include medications, lifestyle

changes, therapy, and support for caregivers. Dementia currently has no recognized cure.

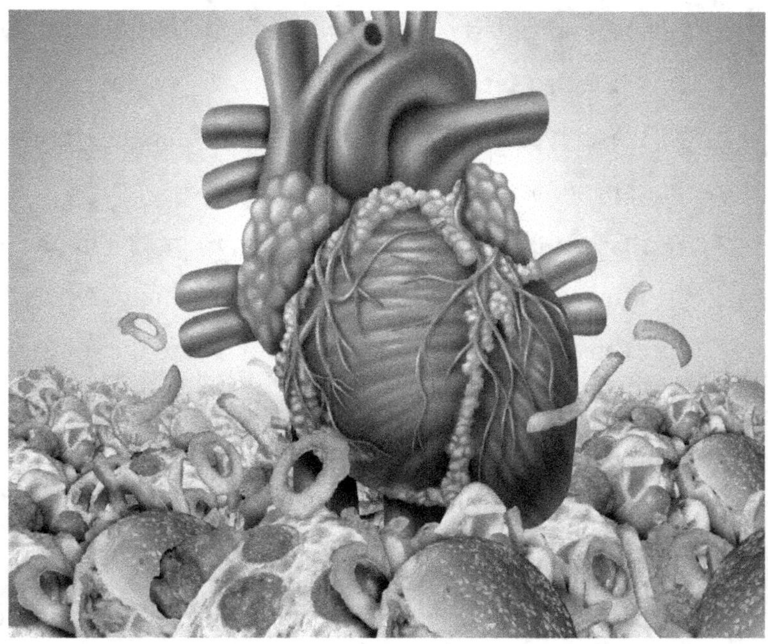

3. **Heart disease**: Heart disease in elderly people is a term used to describe any condition that affects the heart, such as coronary artery disease, congestive heart failure, or an irregular heartbeat. It occurs when the heart is unable to pump enough blood to meet the body's needs, often due to a buildup of plaque in the arteries. The risk of developing heart disease increases with age due to changes in blood vessel structure and the accumulation of fat, cholesterol and other substances in the arteries. Elderly people are also more likely to have other conditions that increase their risk

of heart disease such as high blood pressure, high cholesterol, diabetes, and obesity. Symptoms of heart disease in elderly people can include chest pain, shortness of breath, fatigue, and dizziness. Treatment for heart disease typically includes lifestyle changes, medications, and in some cases, surgery.

4. **Falls**: Falls are a leading cause of injury in the elderly, leading to broken bones, head injuries and even death. To prevent falls, it is important to keep the home free of clutter, secure items that may cause tripping, and wear non-slip shoes.

5. **Cognitive Decline:** Cognitive decline is the loss of mental function and can be prevented by staying mentally active and engaging in activities such as reading, puzzles, and social activities.

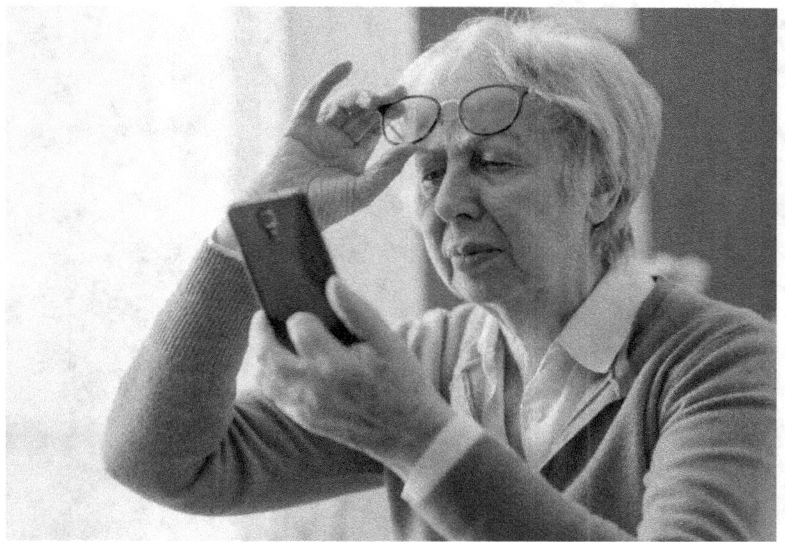

6. **Vision Loss:** Vision loss is common in the elderly and can be prevented by having regular eye exams and wearing sunglasses when outdoors.

7. **Hearing Loss**: Hearing loss is also common in the elderly and can be prevented by having regular hearing tests and avoiding loud noises.

8. **Urinary Incontinence**: This is the inability to control bladder and bowel movements and can be prevented by staying active, doing Kegel exercises, and avoiding certain foods and drinks.

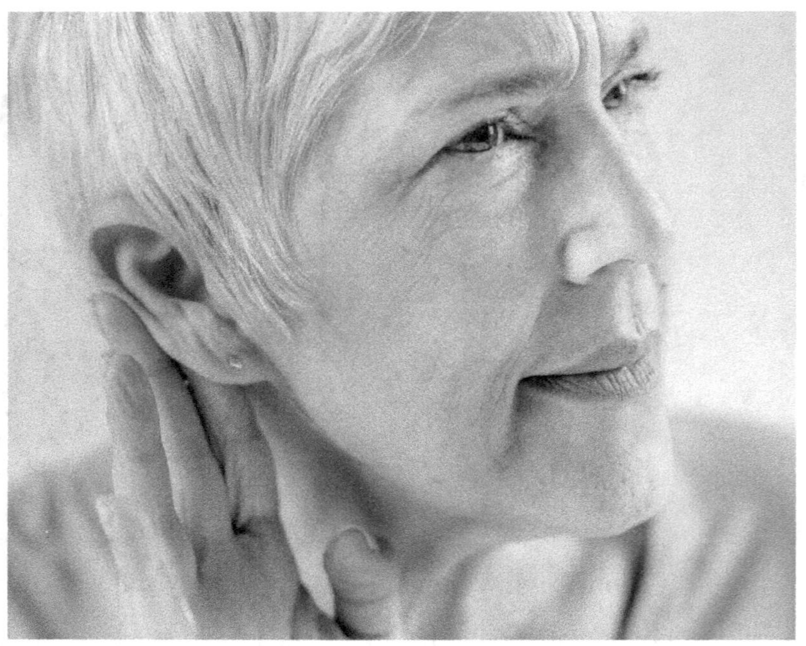

9. **Pressure Sores:** Pressure sores are caused by skin breakdown due to prolonged pressure on the skin. To prevent them, it is important to keep the skin clean and dry, and to reposition the body regularly.

10. **Depression**: This is a common condition in the elderly that can be prevented by engaging in social activities, staying connected to family and friends, and seeking professional help if needed.

11. **Diabetes:** Diabetes is a condition in which the body cannot properly use the sugar it gets from food. It can be prevented by eating a healthy diet, exercising regularly, and maintaining a healthy weight.

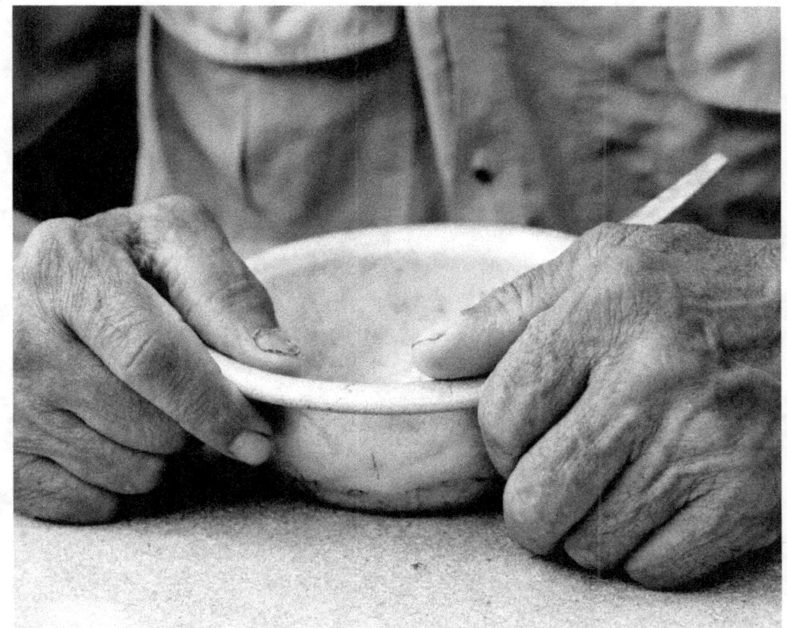

12. **Malnutrition:** Malnutrition is a common problem in the elderly and can be prevented by eating a balanced diet and taking nutritional supplements as needed.

13. **Dehydration:** Dehydration is a condition in which the body does not have enough fluids and can be prevented by drinking plenty of fluids and avoiding alcohol.

14. **Constipation**: Constipation is a common problem in the elderly and can be prevented by eating plenty of fiber-rich foods, drinking plenty of fluids, and exercising regularly.

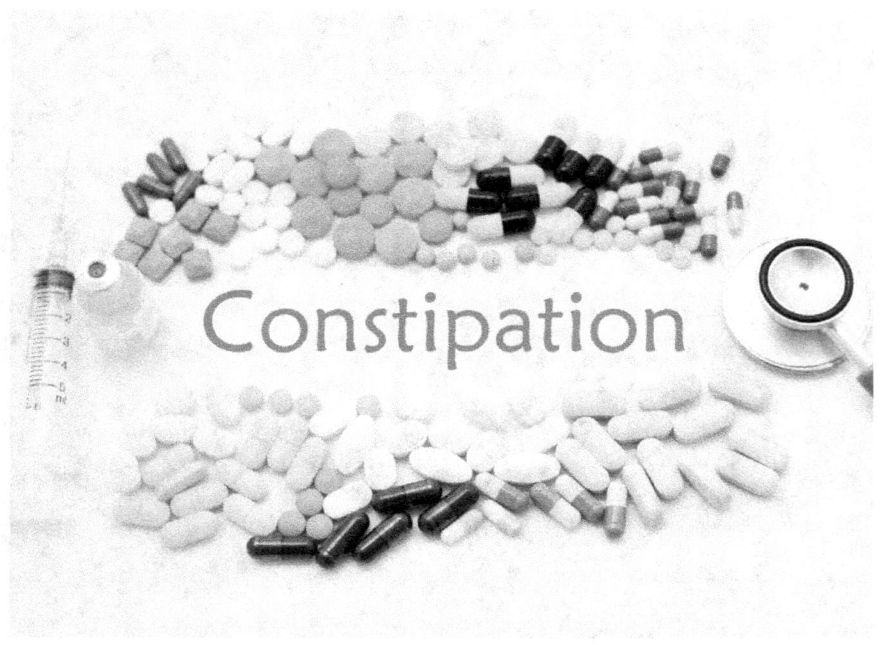
Constipation

CONCLUSION

Age Slower, Live Longer: A Guide to Longevity and Vitality is a helpful resource for anyone looking to incorporate healthy lifestyle changes into their life. The various topics covered throughout the guide provide readers with the knowledge and understanding needed to make positive changes that can lead to a healthier, longer life.

The guide outlines the importance of exercise, proper nutrition, stress management, and sleep. Through these topics, readers can gain an understanding of how to incorporate these elements into their daily life to improve overall health and wellbeing. The book also discusses the importance of maintaining a positive attitude and outlook, as well as the benefits of social interaction.

Overall, Age Slower, Live Longer: A Guide to Longevity and Vitality is an excellent resource for anyone looking to make positive changes in their life. It provides clear, concise information about the various elements that contribute to health and longevity. By following the advice outlined in the guide, readers can gain a better understanding of how to live a healthier, longer life. While there are no guarantees that one will remain healthy and age slowly, following the guidelines can certainly improve the chances of doing so. To ensure the best possible chance of living a longer, healthier life, it is important to take an active role in one's own health and wellbeing. Age Slower, Live Longer: A Guide to Longevity and Vitality can help readers do just that.

www.ingramcontent.com/pod-product-compliance
Lightning Source LLC
Chambersburg PA
CBHW070754250726
48662CB00004B/1803